KICKSTART FAT LOSS

TRANSFORM YOUR BODY AFTER 40 AND RECLAIM YOUR POWER

MELISSA NEILL

Difference Press

Washington DC, USA

Published 2024

DISCLAIMER

Cover Designer: Jennifer Stimson

Editor: Madeline Kosten

Front cover photo courtesy of Laura Skye

Back cover photo courtesy of Creative Instincts

To my dear mother, Joan Freeland, who taught me so many things about life – determination, not to let society dictate your life, and to find strength in the face of adversity.

CONTENTS

SHOULD LOSING WEIGHT REALLY BE THIS HARD?

ach morning, Linda stood in front of her closet. The doors wide open, she did the infamous Shirt Shuffle. Considering the weather outside and how comfortable she wanted to be, she flipped through her outfit options, methodically walking her fingers across the hangers, from left to right, whittling down her options.

Each blouse, sweater, and skirt that she passed over received a similar verdict: too small, too tight, too revealing.

She was fifty-two, a mother and wife, and constantly taunted by the clothes in her closet. Sure, the complexities of midlife had started to get to her, but she was surviving. Right?

When she finished running her fingers down the line of shirts, still nothing picked out, she did the Shirt

Shuffle again, this time right to left, hoping maybe something would pop out that she hadn't seen the first time. But nothing did. There were a handful of blouses that she wore frequently, so she settled for her favorite, knowing it would make her comfortable. In other words, it would help her survive the day without obsessing over her weight.

Sadly, Linda's story isn't just about numbers on a scale. It's about the emotional weight she carried – the loss of confidence, the disconnection from the vibrant woman she used to be. She'd look in the mirror and barely recognize herself, wondering where that spark had gone.

One day, as she struggled to zip up yet another pair of jeans, Linda reached her tipping point. She faced a decision that many of us have grappled with: should she simply go out and buy new clothes to accommodate her changing body, or was it time to make a real change?

Oh, that phrase, "real change." She knew what it meant – training, hard work, grueling hours, and most likely a dietary change. But she couldn't bear to think of the specifics. Instead, that phrase, "real change," became the monster in her closet. It sounded scary, out of reach.

The impact of her weight gain reached far beyond her wardrobe. Linda found herself with less energy to keep up with her daughter, Zoe. Family bike rides and playground visits, once a source of joy, now left her feeling exhausted and discouraged. She started avoiding the camera during family gatherings, not wanting to immortalize this version of herself in photos.

Linda's struggle wasn't for lack of trying, though. Like so many, she had attempted various diets and exercise routines over the years. Each time, she'd start with enthusiasm, only to find herself back where she began, feeling more frustrated and defeated than ever. The cycle of hope and disappointment had taken its toll on her mental state.

Balancing family responsibilities with self-care seemed like an impossible task. As a dedicated mother and wife, Linda often put her own needs last. The guilt of taking time for herself warred with her desire to be healthy and present for her family. It's a dilemma many women face – how do we care for ourselves without feeling like we're neglecting our loved ones?

Deep down, Linda knew something had to give. She was tired of feeling tired. Tired of avoiding mirrors and cameras. Tired of the internal battle every time she got dressed. Most of all, she was tired of not feeling like herself.

It wasn't just about looking better in clothes or seeing a lower number on the scale. Linda yearned to feel strong again, to have the energy to fully engage with her family, to rediscover the confidence that had gradually slipped away. She wanted to be a role model for her daughter, showing Zoe that it's never too late to prioritize your health and well-being.

Linda was determined to drag that monster out of her closet and finally commit to not just real change, but to living life on her terms – healthier and happier.

YOU'RE NOT ALONE

Maybe you, like Linda, have stood in front of your closet doing the Shirt Shuffle just fast enough to avoid that monster lurking in your closet. Maybe you've avoided social outings, shied away from the camera, or felt that twinge of guilt when you can't keep up with your kids like you used to.

I hear it all the time. I say that not to diminish your concerns, but to let you know that you are not alone. I have worked with countless women over forty, and you'd be shocked at how many women share your frustrations – clothes no longer fitting, feeling disconnected from your own body.

Remember how easy it used to be to drop a few pounds? Maybe you'd cut back on desserts or hit the gym a bit more, and voila! But now? It feels like your body is playing by a whole new set of rules. You're doing everything "right," yet the scale won't budge. It's maddening, isn't it?

And the energy drain – oh, I hear you on this one. Remember when you could work all day, hit the gym, and still have energy for a night out? Now, just getting through your to-do list feels like climbing Everest.

The most frustrating part? Those diets that used to work like magic now seem to have lost their sparkle. Low-fat, low-carb, juice cleanses – you name it, you've probably tried it. And when they don't work, it's easy to feel like you're doing something wrong.

All of this takes a toll. The frustration, the hope-lessness – it creeps into every part of your life. The monster of "real change" lurks in your closet when you're simply figuring out what to wear each morning. Your confidence takes a hit. Relationships can strain under the weight of your dissatisfaction. I've been there, feeling like I was letting myself and everyone else down.

But here's the thing: understand that you're not alone; this is a shared experience! Understanding this is the first step towards change. We're in this together, and together, we can find a way forward.

UNDERSTANDING THE CHANGES IN
YOUR BODY

What most people seem to mention yet never seem to really zone in on is that your body completely changes after forty. You're playing a new game, and no one lets you in on the rules. If you're lucky, you have a great primary care physician you see for routine check-ups, or perhaps you keep up to date on health articles to better understand your changing body, so you might have some insight. But if you're like any other woman over forty I know, how could you possibly have the time? It seems like to truly understand what happens to the female body as it ages, you need a degree and all the time in the world to do research. The worst part is that, once you know what's happening under the hood, everything starts to make a lot more sense.

First up, hormones. Oh boy, do they love to shake things up! As we age, our estrogen and progesterone levels start to dip. It's like someone's slowly turning down the volume on these crucial hormones. And your thyroid? It might be feeling a bit sluggish too. All this hormonal hocus-pocus has a direct impact on how your body functions.

Now, let's talk metabolism. Remember when you could eat a slice of cake without it showing up on your belly the next day? Those were the days! After forty, our metabolism decides to take things slow. Like, really slow. It's like it's on permanent vacation mode. And here's the kicker – your body becomes a champion at storing fat, especially around your midsection. That's right, hello, menopausal belly!

So, why do all those diets that used to work now feel like exercises in futility? It's simple – they're not designed for your new body's chemistry. It's like trying to use an old map in a newly renovated city. You'll just end up lost and frustrated.

This is why a cookie-cutter approach just doesn't cut it anymore. Your body is unique, and it needs a tailored strategy. We need to work with your changing hormones, not against them. We need to outsmart that slowing metabolism and kick it back into gear.

IT'S TIME TO BREAK THE CYCLE

With every morning that passes, every shirt that no longer fits, and the mounting frustration you feel, you try to shove that monster of "real change" a little deeper in your closet, making it harder to get out. But let's face it, you've been on this ride for far too long, and it's time to change.

This is why I do what I do. I know you're too busy to go out and get that exercise science degree or do hours of research. I know, because I, too, used to do the

Shirt Shuffle. I, too, used to have a monster hidden way in the back of my closet. So, I went out and did the hard work, so you won't have to.

Within this book, you'll find my years of experience helping fabulous women over forty finally achieve the bodies of their dreams – and keep them.

No more Shirt Shuffles.

No more outfits that no longer fit.

No more monsters in the closet.

I'm talking about real, sustainable change that helps you float back to the top, so to speak. Change that will help you recognize that gorgeous face in the mirror again. Change that will leave you feeling comfortable in whichever top you pull out of the closet again. Change that will give you the boost you need to do the activities you used to love doing. Change that will leave you with the energy to spend time with your kids or go for that meal out with your friends. Not only will you enjoy a night out without worrying about the extra calories consumed, but you will also go on vacations again, confident in the swimwear you put on.

It's all about working smarter, not harder. We're talking strength training to fire up that sluggish metabolism and nutrition plans that balance our hormones. No more one-size-fits-all solutions!

Here's the deal: our bodies have unique needs now, and it's time our fitness and nutrition plans reflect that.

We're not trying to turn back the clock here. We're embracing where we are and making the most of it

This isn't about drastic changes that leave you feeling deprived. It's about sustainable, long-term strategies that fit into your life. Because let's face it, we've got enough on our plates without adding complicated diet rules to the mix.

Are you ready to break free from the cycle and start seeing real, lasting results? Let's do this!

2

THE ROAD TO FITNESS IS PAVED
WITH DETERMINATION

Through my childhood and my pre-teen years, I was fit. I was an athletic, sporty child; I did ballet and gymnastics. This passion for movement started early, influenced by my unique upbringing.

Born in the UK in 1967, I spent my early years in Ghana where my mom had moved us shortly after I was born. Life in Ghana was good – we had a big house, and I even became bilingual, speaking both English and Twi, one of the local languages. I was always on the move, playing with other kids and staying active in the warm African sun.

When I was six, we moved back to the UK. It was a big change, and suddenly I was different from the other kids. The more "polite" kids would ask questions like, "Why are you black and your mum is white?" The meaner kids would call me "half-breed," the n-word, and the p-word, an ethnic slur used in the UK. Once, the racist national front held a meeting in our school building, and I was scared to death walking home. To stick together, all the black students decided we should walk home together for protection.

Additionally, growing up with a single mom wasn't easy, but she was determined and strong. On a meager teacher's salary, she struggled to put food on the table and buy new clothes for me, a big point of shame for my mother. She was mortified when she saw my overly short jeans in a school photo, after she couldn't find a new pair for me.

And the challenges kept coming. As a white single mom to a black child, some kids even said my mom must have been a prostitute to have slept with a black man. She faced many difficulties, from finding a place to live to getting a mortgage, but she never gave up. Watching my mom persevere taught me the power of determination – a lesson that would serve me well in my fitness journey years later.

Growing up in the UK as a black child in the 1970s was tough, but through it all I thought back to my childhood in Ghana, when I was always on the move with other kids outdoors, and in the UK, I too found comfort in sports and dance. Being active helped me fit in and gave me confidence.

As I entered my teen years, my focus shifted. I discovered music and boys, and taking care of myself went out the window. You could say I became a bit of a wild child, hitting the clubs and leaving my sporty days behind.

And then I got pregnant when I was eighteen, and fitness took a backseat to motherhood. Things stayed that way for a while, which was fine because I was still slim. Admittedly, I was one of those annoying people you hear about having a baby at a young age who quickly bounce back into shape. I didn't have any problems getting the baby weight off. When I met my ex-husband in my mid-twenties, I was still in good shape, and I stayed that way without much effort.

As I got into my thirties, I started to want to address my health and get into fitness. That was around the time I did start to see my body change, and while I wanted to make healthy changes, I found it increasingly hard to stay at a healthy weight. I realized I had to work a bit harder at my fitness, so I started reading everything I could regarding the best approach to take.

I've always gravitated towards being more muscular than model slim, and I took up strength training at that time. I trained with a competitive body-builder and also ran. The combination of the two worked quite well for me, and my trainer told me I

could get in even better shape if I paid careful attention to what I was eating by weighing and measuring
my food. Of course, I enjoyed a glass of wine and deca-
dent meals on the weekends. When he showed me
what he was eating and recommended it to me – some
combination of chicken breast, broccoli, and rice at
nearly every meal – it looked so unappealing that I
decided I didn't want to eat this way! (Remember, this
was in the nineties; we have so many more options
now.)

When I was thirty-nine, I got pregnant a second
time. Shortly after that, I had my third and youngest
child. I was in a loveless marriage, but I didn't realize it,
and on top of everything else, those weekends of wine
had evolved into a drinking problem. I had stopped
drinking when I was pregnant, but by the time I was in
my early forties, I was hitting the bottle most nights.
(With help from a friend in a 12-step program, I eventually gave up drinking because I realized I was an
addict.)

My problem drinking was masking all the problems that I was going through in my marriage, and
that's when I started really getting out of shape. Once I
stopped drinking for good, I found that I actually did
binge eat at times. Drinking and binge eating were
contributing to my weight problem, and between this
and my failing marriage, my self-image took a hit. I

didn't like how I looked, and I transferred a lot of what was wrong in the marriage onto my appearance.

And then I learned about my husband's infidelity. I was shocked and numb, and when I looked in the mirror, I simply didn't believe I was attractive anymore. I believed I was "over the hill" and that was the reason my now ex-husband had cheated on me – he didn't like my looks or my body shape as I was aging. *How could he, when I didn't either?* I thought.

I began internalizing this pain, thinking my crumbling marriage was my fault. The craziest part is that I was still doing the same exercises that kept me fit in my younger years, but this didn't stop the self-loathing. I could not get in shape, and thought this was simply an inevitable result of growing old, that there was nothing that could be done to help me feel better – both physically and mentally. Daily, this made me question my femininity and attractiveness. I lacked confidence and went into a depression.

A friend told me not to go the route of antidepressants because they can add to addiction issues, but I knew I had to do something. This time, I thought working on my mental health and building confidence was more important than my physical appearance. I remembered how good and confident I was when I had exercised consistently before, so I once again returned to exercise, and I began doing more research on weight loss and exercise for women over forty.

When I started searching menopause and weight loss online, I found a plethora of bad advice, like extreme dieting and extreme fasting. And that's when I realized it – there was a real lack of information for women over forty when it comes to our health! No wonder it seems so hard for us to lose weight and keep it off.

I learned that on average, women over forty gain around twenty-five pounds. I searched YouTube and other social media sites, and realized there wasn't anybody talking about this. Nobody was giving our experience a voice. We were totally in the dark!

At this point in my journey, I took up CrossFit. CrossFit is a difficult combination of gymnastics, powerlifting, and high intensity interval circuit training (HIIT). I went in the morning after dropping my kids off at school and was surrounded by other mothers. It was a very supportive environment. When I first started going, I remember crying outside as I sat in the car from my marriage breakdown, but once I went in and focused, I felt so much better by the end of the class. My endorphins were going, and at forty-nine, I was accomplishing new things that I had never imagined I would, having believed my best years were already behind me.

Despite being athletic when I was younger, I had never done a pull up or pistol squats (which are incredibly difficult) in my life. The CrossFit coach worked with me, and soon, I was doing handstands, push-ups, pull-ups, and was lifting heavy weights. I wasn't as strong as some of the other women in the gym (they were just absolute monsters!) but they inspired me to push myself a little harder. As I watched them, I thought, *I may not be able to go as heavy as them, but I can go a bit heavier.*

Over time, CrossFit helped me build my confidence; I was getting physically stronger and better at doing exercises that it had never crossed my mind to try, much less be successful at. However, CrossFit is competitive – as an older woman learning new things in a competitive environment, I focused more on speed than form and picked up a lot of injuries in the process.

I stuck with CrossFit for about two years, when I met up with a friend of mine, a sports massage therapist who knew me for a long time and had advised me on exercise when I had a period of bad neck and shoulder pain in my mid-forties. When I took up CrossFit, he was quite happy with it at first because he said it would help me build the muscles around the areas that were giving me problems. I did feel better because CrossFit emphasized strength training, which I wasn't doing much of before. I still felt as though I needed to continue running to burn fat, but I was putting on weight. When I saw him again, I was riddled with injuries and he said, "I think it's time to stop CrossFit, Melissa. You should switch primarily to strength training."

With my mental health now in a good place, I started to think about sculpting my body. I was taking more of an interest in my appearance. There was a magazine I used to buy called *Muscle and Fitness Hers* out of the US. I wanted the looks I saw in that magazine; I wanted to be muscular and defined. I thought, *well, if I switch solely to strength training, that's the look I'm going to go for.*

As I entered my fifties, my mindset started to change. This time, I didn't just want to be in good shape, I wanted to be in *great* shape. I moved away from CrossFit and went purely into strength training. I discovered by accident that it was more effective for fat burning than doing cardio. Needless to say, I quit running.

Although I'd been lifting heavy at CrossFit, I was in my fifties when I first started strength training with a trainer who gave me the wrong advice (more on that in the next chapter). After a few months, I ditched him and started writing my own workout programs. My body was changing but it wasn't quite where I wanted to be because I hadn't got the nutrition right. I knew that I needed to intake high levels of protein, but my nutrition had to be precise to get in muscular shape. At that point, I just didn't have it.

Of course, I was gradually changing, but I had this vision about what I wanted to look like – the women in *Muscle and Fitness Hers*, and I wasn't there. I wasn't going to give up pursuing this dream, so I became really determined. When I saw people like Ernestine Shepherd, who is in her eighties and a competing bodybuilder, I thought, *there must be something wrong, she's in her eighties after all and she looks amazing.*

I decided to try my hand at competitive body-building and bikini competitions. I looked for a coach and thought I had found one. She showed me pictures of women who she said she helped get to the stage and it seemed like a good fit for me. Unfortunately, it didn't work out as I had planned. (Again, I'll go into further detail in the next chapter – just know, for now, that my success wasn't a straight line. In fact, there were many obstacles to overcome.)

I was about fifty-two when I cut ties with this coach. Discouraged, I went off the idea of competing at all, but I still wanted to get in the best shape of my life and began really working on myself. I did loads of research and began retraining myself – and it was working. I started improving almost immediately. That was when I really began to learn what fitness and strength training was all about.

I was still interested in bikini competitions, and I went to see a friend compete. It was there that my fire for competitive body building came back. I spent about five weeks working toward a competition on my own, but I wasn't sure I could do it. I needed a coach to guide me, but I needed the right coach. Luckily, I found her in the nick of time. This time, I thought about interviewing her clients, who all sang her praises. She had a record of success with women in their late forties and early fifties, who were usually peri-menopausal. For me, she hit all the marks. We had twelve weeks before the competition, and she guaranteed she could get me to the stage with good nutrition and a solid workout regimen. She noted that I was already in good shape. I was, but I wasn't as muscular and lean as I knew I could be.

I did three competitions in 2019. I came third in the first competition, and I got second and third in the second competition. At the last competition of the year, I won first place! Everything shut down due to the pandemic, but when the world opened back up, I took part in two more competitions with numerous placings in 2021. There are always improvements to make, and if I compete again, I know what changes I'll make to improve my stage physique.

Women are often told that we've got to resign ourselves to a certain physique when we get older, and it's just not possible to get in the kind of shape we want to get into. That is just a myth – one I never believed. I never gave up hope, even though I had setbacks, which sometimes made me question everything. In order to attain my dreams and health goals, I made the necessary sacrifices.

I was not ready to do this when I was in my mid-thirties, but in my late forties, I was ready to make those sacrifices. I had lived my life; I'd done what I wanted to do. I'd been the party girl. It was now time to focus on self-care and getting into great physical shape. It wasn't just about how I looked, it was about feeling good, and this journey has given me confidence in every area of my life. Fitness has helped me achieve everything that I could have possibly imagined.

I even completely changed my career because of fitness.

After having done my initial research into weight loss after forty and realizing how little information there was out there for women, in the summer of 2019, I decided to start my own blog and YouTube channel. Now, that channel has grown to over 300,000 subscribers, with 24 million total views. It just goes to show you the real need for this information!

When I first started my YouTube channel, it was

hard to get viewers interested in my content. But of course, success on YouTube doesn't happen overnight, and I gradually made more and more videos. There was one particular video that was performing really, really well, giving me many new subscribers.

By January of 2020, I was regularly getting a lot of comments and new subscribers, and I knew there had to be something to my video content!

I decided to make regular videos, at least one a week, but even so, I soon realized this simply wasn't enough. Women – especially busy women over forty – needed a blueprint they could follow. When COVID hit and lockdown began, with gym closures and so much time at home, many people began flocking online for assistance with weight loss that they could do from the comfort of their own homes. So, in June 2020, I launched my own fitness and weight loss program called the Six-Week Shred.

The Six-Week Shred was born out of my tiny living room at home. In the UK, we do tend to live in small homes, and right from my living room, with very little equipment – only two dumbbells, a weighted vest, and resistance bands – I started my program. As it happened, the modest equipment was absolutely perfect for the group of women I was trying to market to. Most women forty years and older do want to work out from home and don't own a lot of equipment, so this was ideal for them.

I set about making a program that included weightlifting and HIIT days, as well as a meal plan that women could easily follow. This meal plan involved weighing and measuring your food and eating high protein meals and snacks.

When I launched the program, I held live events to get feedback. To my excitement, it started to sell well, and I had great feedback pouring in, including before and after pictures! When I saw the results I was able to help women achieve during the program, I knew I was on to something.

By July 2021, I'd moved from content creation as a side hustle into my full-time job. Since then, I've launched numerous programs that can help solve the problems women are having with weight loss. In January 2022, I took my programs to the next level by launching my own unique app called Body by Bikini, available on the App Store and Google Play. As I write this, I've had over 40,000 app downloads and have sold over 10,000 programs.

It is still amazing to me to see how something I created – born out of frustration at not seeing health information for women over forty or going through menopause – has grown to become an incredible community dedicated to helping women achieve better health. On my YouTube channel, I feel that women now have all the information they need to follow the right path when it comes to fitness and weight loss for women over forty, and now I get to bring this information to you in the form of a book!

Now, I don't have to work a job that I don't want; I can make a living out of my passion. I'm happy to give up junk food, not drink alcohol, and not have refined sugar. I'm happy to stick strictly to a meal plan because my body feels great. I met the love of my life in 2017, and we are still together. I attribute this to the newfound confidence I had as a result of my body transformation, which affected every aspect of my life. I have better relationships with my friends and family too. You cannot overestimate how much improving your health is going to enhance every aspect of your life. I'm a different person than the person I was in my late forties, both inside and out. And this can be a reality for you too!

This book will show you how to get started. But remember – it's not an easy road, and you could fail if you don't follow the process I am going to outline for you. I had two and a half years of failure, but you can learn from my mistakes by reading this book.

3

YOUR WEIGHT LOSS JOURNEY
STARTS NOW

Through my transformation and weight loss journey, I experienced a lot of failure, but I believe that it was an important part of why I have success now. I experienced everything that every woman over forty goes through in terms of doing the wrong things to get in shape. I've done them all myself. A lot of women will look at my before and after pictures on social media and say, "Oh, doesn't she look great? She's gone from point A to point B."

But it's not all smooth sailing, especially as you age. In my journey, there were a lot of ups and downs, and what you don't see on social media is that a journey like mine can take quite a long time if you don't follow the right protocol, especially for women over forty.

TRIAL AND ERROR

I've got a background in running, and in my thirties, running worked brilliantly for me. At first, I could see that I was losing body fat, but when I hit my mid-forties, I started gaining weight, despite running about twenty miles a week. I couldn't understand it, but I soon learned running really isn't a good idea for women over forty. It's bad on your joints, and it makes us really hungry, so we end up eating more. I could get away with running in my younger days. I thought, *well, I can eat what I like if I run. I'm putting myself basically into a calorie deficit.* But it just doesn't work like that for older women.

As I mentioned, I also did CrossFit. Yes, I got fitter and stronger. On the surface, you would think that was perfect, and I did learn valuable skills there. But, at the time, what I wasn't doing was combining that workout with the right nutrition.

Intermittent fasting was another failure; I did that for eighteen months, which is quite a substantial amount of time to do something when you're not seeing results. I wasn't losing weight or building muscle. There's such powerful information on the internet, especially on YouTube, but what you will notice is most of the people promoting things like intermittent fasting are actually men, and the research on it has been carried out on mice. There are no specific studies on intermittent fasting and fat loss for menopausal women, and there is no clear evidence that intermittent fasting is more effective for weight loss than a caloric deficit. In fact, as I write this, there has been a study carried out with a randomized control trial. Participants practicing calorie restriction lost more weight than those doing time-restricted eating.

When I was intermittent fasting, I was strength training at 6 a.m. and not eating for five hours because I was following the 16 /8 method – sixteen hours without eating and eating for eight. I didn't see good results from my strength training because I wasn't eating carbs prior to lifting weights, which improves your performance. I also wasn't putting my body into protein synthesis, which means that the protein is going to go into your muscle. The optimum time to do this is by consuming protein within an hour or so after strength training. This is particularly important for older women, as it is much harder to build muscle once you hit your forties. Needless to say, I wasn't seeing very good results.

Intermittent fasting doesn't suit some women very well at all, particularly menopausal women, which I now understand but didn't know at the time. Intermittent fasting can also cause stress fat. Stress fat occurs when your cortisol levels are raised. I find that when I go for extended periods without food, I get stressed and extremely hungry. When I was fasting, my cortisol levels were raised and that in turn affected the balance of my hormones. I found I didn't lose any significant amount of weight whilst intermittent fasting and retained a lot of fat around my midsection, which is not healthy. The midsection is where you store visceral fat. If you are doing extreme fasting – like twenty-four hour fasting or having only one meal a day – you may also find that you are going to lose muscle and not gain it. This is disastrous for women over forty and will completely screw your metabolism.

Eventually, I ditched CrossFit and was trying to sculpt my body, and I went through my share of trainers. I worked with a competitive bodybuilder in my mid-thirties, who did wonders for me, so I found another in my forties, but this time, it was a big mistake. He made the classic mistake that male trainers make with older women by suggesting that if I wanted to lose body fat, I should do high reps with light weights. He also didn't school me properly about the amount of protein I should be taking in, even though he, himself, as a bodybuilder, must have been taking in a great deal of protein. To be fair on him, it isn't a personal trainer's role to advise on nutrition, but *all* trainers must understand that nutrition is the missing link when it comes to changing your body shape. No amount of exercise is going to work unless you get your nutrition right. The adage "you can't out train your fork" is so true. And it's where most people fall down, including me. Through trial and error, I learned that these, and the many mistakes I made before, were holding me back from reaching my goals.

PLOTTING MY OWN JOURNEY

After my failures, I decided to write my own food and workout plans. I met someone at the gym who knew a bit about weight training and got him to help me. Although his plans were made mostly for men, they worked really well for women too and included strength training four times a week, with one HIIT session per week. When I started implementing this training plan, I did make progress, but I was not yet at the point of eating the way I should have been, so I wasn't seeing the results I longed for.

While I was doing all this strength training, a friend mentioned that I should do bikini competitions. She had done one and showed me some pictures of her posing in a sparkling bikini. I didn't know what was involved, but I liked the look of getting on stage in a sparkling bikini and putting myself through the challenge of getting my body in shape. Because I like the muscular look and fitness model magazines, it was always in the back of my mind as something to work towards, but at that point, I couldn't quite see how I was going to get there. Physically, my body wasn't anywhere near that shape, and I still had a lot more body fat to lose. I also wasn't building enough muscle because I just didn't have the right nutrition or approach.

Like I mentioned earlier, at this point, I decided to hire myself a coach to take me to the stage. I had this idea the sparkling bikini was calling me, and I just felt that it was my destiny. But of course, what happened was that she just screwed up royally. I filed this away as a lesson learned – in the future, I needed to do research on any coach.

If you're hiring a coach, you need to actually speak to their clients. The coach I hired bamboozled me with pictures of women who may not have even been clients or perhaps she just helped them with posing and hadn't actually helped them with nutritional training. She had a boyfriend, who was there when I went to have a meeting with her, and in hindsight, it was obvious that she was under pressure to secure me as a client. (I later found out that they were con artists.)

I took her as a coach despite these red flags, and she put me on a low-calorie diet, which was just not suitable for somebody going to stage; she should have had me on higher calories and higher carbs to build my muscle. She also tried to sell me different things like t-shirts and extra training sessions; I was paying through the nose for coaching, and she kept pressuring me to buy more and more stuff. She soon started pressuring me into buying performance enhancing drugs (an illegal fat burner called Clenbuterol). I was determined to compete naturally, and to this day remain a completely natural athlete, so this is when I knew I had to cut my losses. I fired her as my coach and started to give up hope that I was ever going to go to competition. I was discouraged, believing that the only way to stage was to cheat and take performance enhancing drugs, but I now know that isn't true. With the right techniques, you can get to stage and be completely drug free.

ON MY OWN AGAIN

I started to do my own research about nutrition, but I put the whole idea of competing on the back burner because I just thought I had to go to extreme lengths to be able to do it, and I didn't believe I could. I continued to go to the gym because it worked so well for my mental health. When my marriage ended, it kept me on an even keel.

There was a woman at the gym who was much younger than me and getting ready to compete. She wasn't working with my former coach, but she had a friend who was helping her out. I'd already been working on myself for quite some time. Despite the changes I made, I still wasn't in the shape that I dreamed of.

I went to see her compete, and I saw the other female competitors. Some had beach bodies, and some were muscular. When I saw the muscular women, I knew that's what I wanted and after seeing my friend get so far on her own, I decided to book a show in October 2019. I soon realized when I was only twelve weeks away from the competition, that I *still* didn't have the knowledge and experience a coach would, and without one, I could not move forward.

Most bikini competitors have what are called "prep coaches," and I decided to give finding one another try. This time, I decided I was going to interview more than one, and I would ask to speak to three of their clients. They all welcomed me to do so, but there was one woman who I particularly hit it off with.

When I got on the call and told her about my bad experience with the last coach she said, "You don't need to take drugs. What you need to do is have a really good nutrition and workout plan in place."

I told her I had twelve weeks to get ready for the show, and she told me that she would help me in that time. I was worried about my small shoulders, which someone else had pointed out, and she reassured me that judges weren't looking for shoulders – they were looking for glutes and legs. She assured me that I was in good shape and had obviously done quite a bit of work on myself.

With her guidance, I went on a five-meal-a-day-plan. Within weeks, I could see a transformation by just switching up my food; I learned so much from working with her because she's coached women my age. This made a real, lasting difference.

I had my first competition season in 2019. In my first show, I placed third in the over forty-five bikini category, and in the second show, I placed second. My coach thought I should have had first place, but bikini competitions can be very political. At certain shows, there can be plenty of nepotism –that and women who take performance-enhancing drugs can put you at a disadvantage. Regardless, I was elated. I'd made many sacrifices, like spending less time with my kids, so that I could prepare for these shows. This success gave me the confidence to go on and improve every aspect of my life.

THINKING FOR YOURSELF

When doing a competition, you have to have a really strong mind and focus on yourself. The same goes for anyone's mindset when embarking on a weight loss journey. What I learned is not to worry about what anyone else is doing. Anything can happen, as long as you've done your absolute best to train as hard as you can and eat the right way.

I went to a show in November 2019, where I came first in the over forty-five fitness model category. That was the pinnacle for me; I just worked my ass off to get into shape. When I first decided to enter shows, I just thought: *Well, as long as I can get on stage, and look as though I look like I belong, that's all I want.* But by the time I went to the show in November 2019, I wanted to win. I wanted to be the best. I had the ability to do that because I just grew in confidence so much. I was fifty-two years old.

In hindsight, my failure was also a lack of confidence before I started in the competitive bodybuilding world. Whether bodybuilding or just losing a few pounds, this belief in yourself above all is crucial. You have to believe that you can do it, don't you? If you think you can't do it, you're not going to do it. So, you have to believe you can.

This is not going to happen overnight – you have to have the patience to be able to do it. You'll also need to block out things that people say because they will have opinions, telling you what you should and shouldn't do to get fit. If you listen to every word, then you wouldn't get anywhere at all. The most important voice to listen to is your own, and that of your coach, if you are working with one you trust. Another mistake I made was trying to incorporate too many strategies, so ignore all the noise, and focus on one strategy. This way, you're going to get better results.

4

HORMONAL HARMONY: YOUR
MIDLIFE SURVIVAL GUIDE

When Rebecca first came to me, she was forty-eight and had unpredictable mood swings, stubborn weight gain (especially around her midsection), and energy levels that mimicked the lows and highs of a roller coaster. Yup, Rebecca was experiencing the classic signs of perimenopause. Let's just put it this way, her physical life was miserable. And it showed.

"I've always been able to manage my weight," she told me, her voice dripping with exasperation. "But now? No matter what I do, nothing works."

Let's face it, perimenopause can feel like your body's gone rogue. It's not just in Rebecca's head (or yours). During this time, your hormones – especially estrogen and progesterone – start to fluctuate wildly.

It's like a hormonal roller coaster, and it affects everything from your mood to your waistline.

For Rebecca, and many women like her – women like *you* – these hormonal changes wreaked havoc on her body composition. The weight she used to be able to lose easily was now stubbornly sticking around, particularly around her midsection. This isn't just annoying – it's also linked to increased health risks. But here's the kicker: the strategies that worked in your twenties and thirties often fall flat during this hormonal shift.

Initially, Rebecca tried her old go-to methods: cutting calories drastically and spending hours on the treadmill. Sound familiar? But instead of shedding pounds, she found herself more exhausted and frustrated than ever. That's when she realized she needed a different approach – one that worked with her changing hormones, not against them.

THE TRANSFORMATION PROCESS

Finally, Rebecca learned about the huge impact our hormones have on weight and body composition, especially during perimenopause. It was a light bulb moment for her. It finally made sense that those strategies that worked like magic for her in her twenties and thirties fell flat when her hormones decided to throw a party.

So, Rebecca joined my program, and we took a hormone-aware approach to fitness and nutrition. And let me tell you, it was a game-changer for her – just like it will be for you!

As she progressed through the program, Rebecca started noticing some big changes to her body, particularly around her middle. That stubborn belly fat that had been clinging on for dear life? It started to melt away. And this wasn't just about looking good in her jeans (although that was a nice bonus). Rebecca learned how important it was for her overall health to reduce that abdominal fat.

The best part? Rebecca's energy levels skyrocketed. She no longer felt like she needed to mainline coffee just to make it through the day. She started sleeping better at night and waking up feeling ready to take on the world.

The impact on Rebecca's overall well-being was huge. She felt like she'd regained control over her body. She understood what was happening and had the tools to manage it. And let me tell you, that knowledge alone was empowering as hell.

You see, perimenopause doesn't have to derail your health and fitness goals. It's not about fighting against your hormones but working with them. With the right approach, you can not only manage these changes but also thrive during this time.

UNDERSTANDING YOUR HORMONES: THE PROCESS OF PERIMENOPAUSE

Like Rebecca, you need to know what's happening to your body as you age, so you can understand why it can be so difficult to lose weight or get in shape. There's a shift in balance in your hormones, which has a big impact on your ability to lose weight, and your metabolism changes as you get older.

When you get to your thirties and forties, you begin to experience changes in your levels of progesterone and estrogen. For example, many women can experience estrogen dominance. Women of African and Asian heritage often get fibroids, which can be caused by estrogen dominance. In that same period of time, you tend to get symptoms similar to PMS, but they're much more pronounced.

Then during late perimenopause – your late forties and fifties – your estrogen and progesterone actually depletes, and this has an effect on the hormones of your adrenal glands (cortisol and adrenal hormones), as well as the pancreas and thyroid gland.

When your body is out of balance, it begins to store fat. When you try and do the things that you used to do when you're younger to lose weight, it no longer seems to work because your hormones are out of sync. They're changing far faster than they did in puberty. So, you can have mood swings, hot flashes, and anxiety, among many other symptoms. For example, women tell me, "I just don't feel like doing anything." That feeling is completely normal because it's not about a lack of motivation – your body is truly changing.

Some women are affected by this change more than others. Some say they have a really smooth transition, and they don't feel anything at all. For others, it's changed their whole lives – they're very anxious, they can't sleep, and they feel physically drained. With little energy, it's no wonder so many women in peri-menopause don't feel like exercising.

DEFINING MENOPAUSE

Menopause is when your period finally stops, and although your hormones have been depleting, by this point, they're actually settling down and you may start to feel better as your symptoms improve, but for some women symptoms continue well into post menopause. Of course, because of depleting estrogen and progesterone, you're going to have challenges around weight loss. At this point, you're going to experience aging changes, rather than hormonal changes.

Post-menopause begins one year after menopause and lasts for the rest of your life. It takes about two years to adjust to these lower levels of hormones. At this stage, you can't lose weight as easily as you did when you were younger; in fact, it takes longer. Even if you're doing everything correctly, you have to accept that your body isn't going to lose body fat in the way that it did when you were younger. I see this in myself because I'm a competitive bodybuilder, and it takes me longer to get into stage condition compared to someone in their twenties. But you have to accept that your body has changed, and work with what you have.

COMBATING HORMONAL CHANGES WITH FOOD

Many of us can get something called adrenal fatigue when your hormones are out of kilter due to raised cortisol levels. As you get older, you've got to be careful not to put too much stress on your body. You can attempt to eat the right foods, but there are certain foods that are going to exacerbate that hormone imbalance. High fructose corn syrup, refined sugars, trans fats, and processed foods are going to be bad for your hormones. If you eat a healthy, whole foods diet, it will make your perimenopause and menopause symptoms better.

Typically, women whose hormones are out of balance often get blamed for not losing weight. People (including doctors) will say, "All you need to do is be in a calorie deficit." I also know health coaches who do this; when they give a client a diet plan and the client comes back and nothing has changed, the coach is shocked. Well, that's because the client might be in a calorie deficit, but they're eating the wrong types of foods; you have to eat for your hormones. Some of the things that can balance your hormones are good fats, like avocado, olive oil, oily fish, nuts, and nut butters. Protein will also help; in fact, you're going to have to eat more protein than you're used to eating ever in your life. Women should be eating roughly 1 gram of protein per pound in body weight. For women over 170 lbs, they should be eating 1g of protein per pound of their ideal body weight. To consume this much protein, it means women must eat protein at every meal and snack.

Doing this keeps you satisfied, as it takes your body longer to break down protein than other macronutrients, like carbohydrates and fats. This will give you fat burning capabilities that you need to increase your metabolism.

You have to be careful that you're not cutting out carbohydrates. If you're suffering from adrenal fatigue and you're not eating carbohydrates, it's going to make things even worse. You see, your body needs the energy that it gets from carbohydrates to restore itself. Carbo-hydrates are important for things like brain function, but you shouldn't be eating things like fries, chips, or donuts. Instead, you need rice, potatoes, oatmeal, fruits, and vegetables. You certainly shouldn't fear carbs; I get stage lean by eating carbohydrates.

EXERCISING TO HELP BALANCE OUT HORMONES

In terms of exercising for hormones, you can get it completely wrong because nobody tells you how to approach exercise in menopause. When you start working out, you think, *I did whatever it was exercise class or fitness method back in the day, and it really worked, so I'm going to do it again.* Perhaps you used to do BodyPump, Orangetheory, or Pilates but you soon find that it doesn't work for your body anymore.

As I described earlier, your hormones are out of balance, and your reduced levels and the aging processes cause you to lose muscle. So, some types of cardio activity no longer work anymore.

I was doing a lot of running because running really worked in my younger days, and I thought it was all I needed to burn fat. I wouldn't blame anyone thinking that because cardio (including running) does work well when you're younger, but as we age, running puts too much stress on our bodies and will cause us to lose muscle, which can actually make things worse. I gained weight when I took up running again because it was putting too much stress on my body and reducing my muscle. You will find that when you're starting to go through perimenopause, all that cardio is going to reduce your muscle. In this stage in life, muscle is the one thing you cannot afford to lose because you are losing muscle at a rate of just under 1 percent per year. Muscle is important, as muscle will help you burn more calories even at rest. What you need to be doing is the opposite of what you naturally think and that's doing *less* cardio. Often, when women don't see results from the cardio they do, they increase their cardio, but women should be doing the opposite. Instead, women should be pulling back from cardio and turning their attention to strength training.

As you've lost your muscle mass, strength training will increase your basal metabolic rate, in other words, the numbers of calories your burn at rest. You *can* do HIIT but not too much – just fifteen to thirty minutes at a time. If you just keep it to those low levels, it helps burn more fat.

The other good thing that doesn't put any stress on your body and helps you retain muscle is walking. Everyone can walk; it's easy on your joints, unlike running, and it's not going to interfere with your hormones. Some women who come to me are not doing any exercise at all. I start them off with strength training and walking. Walking is still a good cardiovascular exercise, but it's not intense cardio. It's also important to get sleep and rest, and I'll go over both in a little more detail later on in the book. For the days where you're not exercising, walking is absolutely okay.

I know rest is quite difficult for some people. Many women I speak to in the US have very demanding jobs where they work long hours. Around menopause, you may want to reassess your work-life balance and whether or not you're in the right job because burnout can happen easily during perimenopause and menopause. Perhaps you have the stress of looking after elderly parents, or perhaps you've got children, and on top of that, a very demanding job. I know you need to earn money, but perhaps there's a different role you can take on or this may be a good time in life to completely change direction in your work and life. That's what I did, and I wouldn't be talking to you now if I didn't decide at fifty-two to start educating women my age about weight loss.

People come to me because they are interested in (or frankly stressed out about) losing weight. I know this. And I understand why that feels so urgent and important, but my passion in helping women lose weight comes from a deep knowledge that this is going to be important to your overall health, not just your weight loss. The philosophy I am teaching you here on these pages and on my YouTube channel youtube. com/@melissaneill will help you lose weight. If you're really serious about making a change, download my *free* seven-day program on my Body By Bikini app at melissaneill.com/plan. More details can be found in the Gift for Reader page in this book.

I have seen this help literally thousands of women, but if you take it to heart, it will help you make permanent shifts that will serve you for the rest of your life far beyond weight loss. That transition all starts with learning a new (sustainable) way to eat. (And I promise you won't be hungry.)

5

YOUR NEW FOOD PHILOSOPHY

HOW ELSIE STOPPED 'WINE'ING

At forty-four inches, Elsie's waist was the largest it had ever been. As a mother of two daughters, aged twelve and fifteen, Elsie felt a pang of guilt. How could she teach them healthy habits when she couldn't control her own health?

Every night, Elsie found herself reaching for a bottle of wine. It had become her nightly ritual, a way to cope with the stress of her demanding job. One glass turned into two, then three, until the bottle was empty. She knew it wasn't healthy, but it seemed like the only way to unwind.

During the day, Elsie's eating habits were just as chaotic. She snacked often, grabbing whatever was convenient without considering portion sizes or nutritional value. Sweets were her weakness, providing a momentary sugar rush to get through the afternoon slump. But the crash always came, leaving her feeling sluggish and reaching for more unhealthy snacks.

Elsie's unhealthy relationship with food and alcohol was taking its toll. She lacked energy, struggled to keep up with her daughters, and felt disconnected from the vibrant, active woman she used to be. She knew something had to change but wasn't sure where to start.

That's when Elsie discovered my program.

For the first time, she learned about proper portion control and the importance of balanced meals. Instead of mindless snacking, she started eating regular, nutrient-dense meals that kept her satisfied throughout the day.

One of the biggest changes for Elsie was the emphasis on protein. She had always associated protein with bulky bodybuilders, not middle-aged moms. But as she incorporated more protein into her diet, she noticed her energy levels stabilizing and her cravings diminishing.

Even better, our program helped Elsie break her nightly wine habit. (That's a mindset trick I'll cover later, don't worry.) With nutritious dinners and healthy evening snack options, she found she no longer needed alcohol to unwind. The absence of empty wine calories, combined with her new, balanced diet, led to steady weight loss.

As the weeks passed, Elsie's body began to transform. Her waist shrank from forty-four inches to thirty-seven inches, and she lost twenty pounds. Elsie felt stronger, more energetic, and more in control of her life.

Instead of collapsing on the couch after dinner, Elsie now had the energy to engage with her daughters. She played tennis with her youngest, went paddle boarding after arm day (managing an impressive two-mile paddle), and even started joining them on hikes without struggling to keep up.

Perhaps the most touching moment came when Elsie's fifteen-year-old daughter convinced her to wear a bikini – something she hadn't done since she was twenty-nine. Standing on the beach, Elsie realized how far she'd come. Not only had she lost weight and gained muscle definition (her twelve-year-old gleefully pointed out that her mom no longer had a "pancake butt"), but Elsie had also gained confidence and self-respect.

The key to what I taught Elsie was this: your body is a vessel, and you need to keep it fueled properly if you want the ship to keep sailing. You need to learn how to listen to your body, how to fuel it properly for workouts and daily life, and how to find balance in your diet without feeling deprived.

So, with that, let's dig into just how, exactly, you can create a diet that works for you.

A DIET THAT WORKS WITH YOUR HORMONES

Just like I taught Elsie, hormone health is at the heart of the new eating philosophy I'm about to teach you. You need to eat the foods that your body requires for hormone health. Meals that are high in protein help you retain and build muscle, which in turn burns fat, but these meals are also going to help keep you satisfied. Before menopause, you might not have needed as much protein as you do now, but that has all changed and that means you need a new food philosophy. Bodies take longer to break down protein than they do carbohydrates and fats. This means you will burn more calories when you consume protein (compared with carbs and fats) and you won't be as hungry. As a result, you will eat fewer calories in the end even though that's not what we will focus on. Protein is a really important part of making this meal plan work. You need to fuel your body properly in pre-and post-menopause, so that you actually have enough energy to get through the day.

This isn't a low-calorie diet, nor is it low in carbo-hydrates. You need enough energy to fuel your body, and also work out, if you're going to do strength train-ing, which I highly recommend. More protein creates more energy. Strength training creates more muscle. More muscle on your body burns more excess weight. Together, all of this creates a virtuous circle that bene-fits you far beyond weight loss, though that is a great side benefit! You must eat the right foods to help with strength training because it relies heavily on you having enough of the right food in your system to get the proper benefits. As older women, it's actually quite hard to build muscle; in fact, it's harder for you than it is for a young woman or a man the same age as you. This is something I've learned with my own body. When I wasn't fueling my body correctly, I didn't make any progress with strength training, and I don't want this to happen to you. I also found my body burned more calories than ever before when I started incorpo-rating more protein in my diet.

I've laid out a typical nutrition plan for you because I want you to be able to get the most out of strength training, which will help you lose body fat. But you can't lose it by strength training alone. You have to adhere to a specific eating plan to see real bene-fits from strength training.

This meal plan covers all types of diets, whether

you're a vegetarian, a vegan, or a pescatarian. This is a basic plan that has something for everybody. However, if you want a more detailed plan that matches your particular dietary requirements, you can buy a program on my website at melissaneill.com. I've come up with a sample plan for this book, and there are several food choices you can make. For example, I am not entirely plant-based, but I enjoy plant-based foods, and it can be customized to your preferences as well.

LET'S TALK ABOUT PROTEIN

Let's talk more about protein and how that helped Elsie get such great results. If you only get your protein from meat and fish, you'd actually be consuming quite a lot of animal protein throughout the day, so you may want to complement that with some plant-based sources of protein, although you don't have to. Everyone can eat plant-based foods, and I recommend that you try them because they are better for the environment, and I also know some people reading this may feel a bit uncomfortable with the amount of protein in this plan if you're taking it purely from animal sources.

However, plant-based protein sources can also be challenging in their own way. Beans are one such food – you're going to have to eat about nine ounces of beans to equal four ounces of chicken to get your protein in, so you have to think about things in a slightly different way.

Refined sugar, refined carbohydrates, and ultra-processed foods have inflammatory properties, which can especially affect women over forty, so women should try to stay away from alcohol, junk food, and chocolate, for example. The foods in the plan will be anti-inflammatory; therefore, there won't be too many processed foods and those that unbalance your hormones even more.

It's important to try to eat everything on the plan; don't skip meals. Starving yourself can actually damage your metabolism. What you're trying to do with this plan is to speed up your metabolism. Conversely, don't force feed yourself. If you are struggling to get all the food in at first, gradually build up the volume of food. Eating like this may be a struggle, especially if you are someone who has been eating low calories or low carbs previously. If you haven't eaten like this before, you will find you're going to have more energy. There are a lot of meals on this meal plan, but they are small meals throughout the day. If you want to have three meals a day, you could always add two of the smaller meals together, if that's more comfortable for you.

You may even be able to manage your menopause symptoms eating this way because it's a healthy, whole foods diet, which will put you in a good position to be able to do the exercise that I recommend in this book. The main objective is that you're going to lose weight. People find this so surprising because they look at this plan and think, *I'm eating all this food; how can I possibly lose weight?* But remember, we're talking about a body recomposition – building muscle and losing fat all at the same time. For some women, that may mean seeing very little change on the scale. You have to ditch the idea of losing drastic numbers on the scale instantly and focus on waist measurement, how your clothes feel, and how your body looks in before and after photos.

I've seen amazing results eating this way with my own body, and I have seen it happen with the women in my program. I want to share with you now a sample meal plan that is specific to women over forty and fifty so you can see how it might work for you. Remember, the goal isn't to eat exactly this but to match it with your taste and what's available where you live.

Just try and stick to the plan as much as you can. If you do go off, just pick yourself up and get back on track as soon as possible. Whatever you do, don't beat yourself up.

THE SAMPLE MEAL PLAN

This plan is approximately 1,650 calories. Before starting any new diet and exercise program, please check with your doctor and clear any exercise and / or diet changes with them before beginning.

Breakfast Options

Smoked Salmon and Veggie Omelet

Ingredients:

- Oil spray
- Cooked sweet potato (150g / 5oz)
- Broccoli (100g / 3.5oz)
- Smoked salmon (or other cooked or smoked oily fish) – (100g / 3.5oz)
- 2 eggs
- Arugula (for garnish)

Spray non-stick pan with light oil, then add your cooked sweet potato, broccoli, smoked salmon (or other cooked or smoked oily fish), and whisk two eggs and pour over. Cook through and finish under the grill if desired. Serve with arugula (rocket leaves) for garnish.

415 calories, 35g protein, 29g carbs, 15g fat

Tofu and Homemade Baked Beans (Plant-Based/Vegan)

Ingredients:

- Oil spray
- Tofu (100 g / 3.5oz)
- Cooked haricot beans or other beans (100 g / 3.5oz)
- ½ can of blended tomatoes or passata
- Chopped spring onion or scallion
- Garlic paste
- Rye bread (for plating)
- Avocado (for plating)

Cook tofu in pan with light spray oil for 1-2 minutes on each side, put cooked, rinsed haricot (or any other) beans, blended tomatoes, chopped spring onion (scallion), and a teaspoon of garlic paste in separate pan and simmer for 5 minutes. Serve with 1 slice of rye bread and ½ an avocado.

450 calories, 32g protein, 36g carbs, 16g fat

Overnight Protein Oatmeal (Plant-Based/Vegan)

Ingredients:

- Dry weight oatmeal (40g / 1.4oz)
- Almond milk (250mL / 1 cup)
- Protein powder (1.5 scoops)
- Pure almond butter (10g / 1 heaped tsp) or 10g chia seeds
- Blueberries, strawberries, or raspberries (50 g / palmful)

Soak the oatmeal and chia seeds (if added) overnight in your almond milk. In the morning, whisk the protein powder with the almond milk so you have soaked the oats into a paste. Add the protein, mix on top of the oatmeal, then top with your berries, and add almond butter if desired.

430 calories, 39g protein, 36g carbs, 12g fat

Eggs and Protein Shake (Vegetarian)

Ingredients:

- 2 eggs
- 2 slices of wholegrain toast
- Grilled tomatoes and mushrooms
- Protein powder (one scoop)
- Water or unsweetened plant milk

Add your grilled tomatoes and mushrooms to your cooked eggs and serve with your toast. Enjoy with your protein shake, made from a scoop of protein powder mixed with water or unsweetened plant milk.

414 calories, 40g protein, 29g carbs, 13g fat

Lunch Options

Seasoned Protein of Choice with Beans/Lentils and Veggies

Ingredients:

- Skinless chicken, turkey breast, or shrimp seasoned with herbs and/or spices (4oz)
- Sweet potato (140g / 5oz)
- Beans or lentils, drained (50g)
- Low carb vegetables

Enjoy your protein of choice or rotate your choice to keep your lunch option fresh.

418 calories, 44g protein, 35g carbs, 6g fat

Tuna, Baked Potato, and Salad

Ingredients:

- Tuna (110g / 4oz)
- Baked potato (200g / 7oz)
- Lettuce
- Tomato
- Cucumber
- Peppers
- Spring onion

Serve your tuna over your baked potato and make a salad of lettuce, tomato, cucumber, peppers, and spring onion. Add 1 teaspoon of olive oil and lemon juice as dressing for the salad.

408 calories, 36g protein, 44g carbs, 7g fat

Black Bean Burrito Bowl (Plant-Based/Vegan)

Ingredients:

- Black beans (200g)
- Your choice of sliced peppers, raw chili peppers, raw cabbage, raw brussels sprouts, tomatoes, spinach leaves (handful each)
- Half an avocado
- Vegan nutritional yeast (25g / 1 tbsp.)
- Lemon juice

In a bowl, combine your black beans with your choice of peppers, raw chili peppers, raw cabbage, brussels sprouts, tomatoes, spinach, avocado, and sprinkle with vegan nutritional yeast and lemon juice.

452 calories 32g protein, 43g carbs, 8g fat

Veggie "Protein" Crumble Tacos (Plant-Based/Vegan)

Ingredients:

- Textured soy protein or soya meat (soaked in garlic, water, chili pepper flakes) – (50g / 1.7oz)
- Half an avocado
- 6 cherry tomatoes
- 1 spring onion
- Lime juice
- Lettuce leaves
- 1 tortilla

After soaking your soya meat for at least two hours, top your tortilla with the soya protein. Chop the avocado and mix with the lime juice and spring onion. Build your tortilla with lettuce and your soya meat. Serve with the avocado and tomato salsa.

419 calories 37g protein, 19g fat, 22g carbs

Grilled Halloumi Cheese and Peppers, with Kidney Beans and Rice Salad

Ingredients:

- Light Halloumi cheese (60g)
- Red pepper
- Cooked, drained kidney beans (100g / 3.5oz)
- Cooked brown or basmati rice (100g / 3.5oz)
- Tomatoes, cucumber, and green beans
- Lemon or lime juice

Grill or fry Halloumi cheese and red pepper in spray oil. Place cooked, drained kidney beans in a bowl with your brown or basmati rice. Add handful tomatoes, cucumber, and green beans. Mix with lemon or lime juice.

439 calories, 27g protein, 49g carbs, 12g fat

Afternoon Snacks

Protein Berry Shake
Ingredients:

- Protein powder (for whey protein look for an "isolate" and a product without fillers and added carbs or artificial colors) – (1 scoop)
- Strawberries, blueberries, or raspberries (100g / 2 handfuls)
- Unsweetened plant milk (1 cup)

Blend your protein powder, fruit, and plant milk and enjoy!

190 calories, 22 g protein, 17g carbs, 3g fat

Greek Yogurt with 10g Dark Chocolate

Ingredients:

- 0% fat Greek yogurt (150g)
- 70% or higher dark chocolate (10g / 0.5oz)

The creaminess of the yogurt with the decadence of the dark chocolate makes for a fulfilling snack!

175 calories, 17g protein, 9g carbs, 7g fat

Dinner

Ginger and Soy Marinated Fish

Ingredients:

- Salmon, mackerel, or other oily fish (3.5oz)
- Veggies of your choice (e.g. green beans, asparagus, broccoli)
- Spring onion
- Ginger paste
- Unsweetened coconut milk (1 tbsp.)
- Soy sauce (1 tbsp.)
- Fresh chili peppers (optional)
- Konjac noodles (Shirataki noodles) – (optional)

Spread your fish with ginger paste and add spring onion and optional fresh chili peppers. Place in portions and pour on a tablespoon each of unsweetened coconut milk (from the fridge / chiller) and soy sauce. Bake in the oven for ten to fifteen minutes at 350 degrees. Serve with your choice of veggies.

Serve with packet of Konjac noodles (optional), also known as Shirataki noodles (which only have about 9 calories and zero carbs).

241 calories, 24g protein, 4g carbs, 13g fat

Beef and Veggies

Ingredients:

- 3 oz 5% ground beef or sirloin steak (3oz)
- Veggies of choice (e.g. green beans, spinach, or broccoli)

For a simple weeknight meal, enjoy your choice of beef with your favorite veggies.

241 calories 24g protein, 4g carbs, 13g fat

Tofu Cauliflower Curry with Konjac Noodles

Ingredients:

- Tofu (150g)
- Onion (1/2)
- Cauliflower florets (2 to 3)
- Green beans (handful)
- Coconut milk (half a can)
- Peanut butter powder (1 heaped teaspoon)
- Konjac or Shirataki noodles (optional)
- **Spices (1 tsp. each)**:
  - Chili flakes
  - Coriander
  - Cumin
  - Turmeric
  - Garlic paste
  - Ginger paste

In light fry oil, fry half an onion, your tofu, 2-3 cauliflower florets, and green beans. Add your coconut milk and peanut butter powder, and a teaspoon each of your chili flakes, coriander, cumin, turmeric, garlic paste, and ginger paste. Serve with an optional pack of Konjac noodles.

256 calories 26g protein, 9g carbs, 12g fat

Evening or Night-Time Snacks

Watermelon and Nuts

- 100g (3.5 oz) Watermelon or melon (100g / 3.50z)
- Nuts (10g)

85 calories, 2.4g protein, 10g carbs, 4g fat

Dark Chocolate

- 70 % or higher dark chocolate (15g / about one square)

90 calories, 1g protein, 5g carbs, 6g fat

Rice Cakes Spread with Almond Butter

- 2 plain rice cakes
- Almond butter (10g / 1 tsp.)

97 calories, 3g protein, 8g carbs, 6g fat

Optional Pre-Workout Snack

You should eat a meal or snack up to an hour before resistance training and half an hour after resistance training. This is important for muscle building and metabolism. This can be eaten any time of day. If you're not working out, skip this meal.

Rice Cakes with Cream Cheese or Peanut Butter Powder

Ingredients:

- 4 rice cakes
- Low fat cream cheese like Philadelphia Light or peanut butter powder mixed with water (20g / 1 tbsp.)

201 Calories, 12g protein, 31g carbs, 4g fat

Half a Bagel with Cream Cheese or Peanut Butter Powder

Ingredients:

- Half a bagel
- Low fat cream cheese like Philadelphia Light or peanut butter powder mixed with water (20g / 1 tbsp.)
- 201 calories, 12g protein, 31g carbs, 4g fat

Oat Protein Bars

Ingredients:

- Oats (120g / 5.5oz)
- Plant or whey protein powder (4 scoops)
- Unsweetened plant milk (1 cup)

Mix to a sticky consistency, place in a baking dish and bake in the oven for fifteen to twenty minutes at 350 degrees. Cut into four pieces and enjoy one piece.

219 calories, 24g protein, 20g carbs, 3g fat

Maximum total calories: 1664 (depending on choices), up to 157g protein, 152 carbs, and 65g fat

This reduces to 1445 on rest days because you won't eat the pre-workout snack.

TIPS BEFORE STARTING

- Don't go off the plan. Don't have sugar, alcohol, junk food, or chocolate, unless 70 percent dark.
- Don't starve yourself; eat all the meals in the plan if you can, but equally if it's too much at first don't force feed.
- Don't add sauces, mayonnaise, or ketchup, as they are often loaded with calories. However, you can add spices and seasoning.
- Don't let other people persuade you to eat the wrong thing or drink alcohol. Don't go along with the crowd – you are better than that!
- Do start the meal plan once you have done your grocery shopping.
- Do drink at least 64 ounces (2 liters) of

water a day or build up to that if you can't
do that at first.

- Do try to eat *everything* on the plan, even if
you are not hungry. You might struggle to
get everything in, so just build up to it.

IT'S ALL ABOUT TIMING...OR IS IT?

Often when people look at my meal plans like the one
above, they ask when they should eat what. I'm going
to let you in on a secret. I don't believe it matters what
time of day that you eat, but for some people, eating too
close to bedtime can cause digestion issues. Other than
that, it's really not about *when* you eat, it's about *what*
you eat. It's a good idea to taper off on carbohydrates
later in the day, as you'll see in this plan. Carbohydrates are used for energy, and we need less of it as we
go on through the day.

Eating before and after strength training is so
important. I can't stress this enough, and it is where I
went wrong and was the reason I didn't see results at
first. You'll see at the start of the sample plan, there's a
pre-workout snack which can be eaten at any time of
day before you start moving. If you work out in the
morning, eat something with carbohydrates and protein
within an hour of working out. These restore muscle,

and you'll get something called *protein synthesis*, which will help you grow muscle. Remember, you're just putting on muscle that you've lost through the aging process, and that's what's going to help you burn fat.

A lot of women say, "I work out really early in the morning, and I can't eat that early." Well, so do I – I sometimes get up at five and work out at six, but I just ensure that I have something to eat before I do. When I didn't follow this one simple rule, I wasn't seeing the results from my strength training. If you feel you really cannot eat at that time of day, you need to consider whether you should switch your training, because it's just that important. There is a load of scientific evidence that says meals timed before and after training really work, and this is especially important for older women as it is so hard for you to build muscle, so you need to give yourself every opportunity to do this.

Your meal plan and the timing around it is going to be specific to what works for you. Do you have to wake up early for work? Maybe your first meal will be at 4 a.m. Do you find it hard to sleep if you have recently had a meal? Maybe you will stop eating at 6 p.m. Take this sample plan now and customize it before you go shopping, because we are going to give your test meal plan a little, bitty, macro makeover!

If you would like to learn more, go to melissaneill. com/plan.

6

THE MACRO MAKEOVER

Michelle stood at the base of a mountain trail, her hip aching and knees wobbling. The thought of hiking to the top seemed impossible. At home, her clothes felt uncomfortably tight, a constant reminder of her expanding waistline. Menopause had hit her hard, bringing with it joint pain, weight gain, and that stubborn "menopause belly" that seemed impossible to shift.

Every day was a struggle. Simple tasks like climbing stairs or playing with her grandchildren left her winded and in pain. Michelle felt trapped in a body that no longer seemed to be hers. She longed for the energy and vitality she once had, but didn't know how to reclaim it.

Michelle was determined and dedicated as she

completed my eight-week in-app transformation challenge. Though she did a *lot* of work over those eight weeks, her main focus was on macros. If you don't know, macros (short for macronutrients) are the building blocks of our diet. These are proteins, carbohydrates, and fats. Each plays a crucial role in our body's functioning and getting the right balance can be a game changer for your health and fitness goals.

For Michelle, this was a revelation. She discovered the role of each macro: how protein helps build and repair tissues, how carbs fuel our activities, and how healthy fats support hormone production. Michelle began to see food not just as calories, but as fuel with a purpose.

Michelle's approach was methodical. She followed every workout, carefully counted her macros and calories, and made sure she was fueling her body correctly. This wasn't just another diet for her; it was a complete lifestyle overhaul.

What makes Michelle's story particularly inspiring is how she turned her journey into a family affair. Her husband joined her for home workouts, and soon, her adult children were meeting them at the gym for treadmill sessions. Her family's support became a crucial factor in her success.

As Michelle began to understand the importance of macro balance, she saw significant changes in her body and energy levels. The program taught her that it wasn't just about cutting calories, but about providing her body with the right balance of protein, carbohydrates, and fats.

For women over forty like Michelle, understanding macros is crucial. As I explain in this chapter, it's not just about how much you eat, but *what* you eat. By carefully tracking her macros, Michelle ensured she was getting enough protein to build and maintain muscle, enough complex carbohydrates for sustained energy, and enough healthy fats to support hormone balance.

The results spoke for themselves.

"Before long, I began feeling really strong, and the pain in my joints went away," Michelle shared. While the number on the scale was slow to change, her body composition was transforming. She lost three inches off her waist, significantly reducing that stubborn menopause belly.

As Michelle's strength grew, so did her confidence. Though there were days when counting macros felt tedious, and workouts seemed daunting, she persevered, buoyed by the support of her family and the results she saw.

Now, Michelle stands at the top of that mountain trail, taking in the view with a sense of accomplishment she never thought possible. "I am literally able to climb mountains now," she says, the pride evident in her voice.

As we delve deeper into the world of macros in this chapter, I want you to remember Michelle's journey. I want you to understand how implementing the right macro balance can be the key to unlocking your own transformation. Right now, you might be thinking, *yeah right, I don't even know what a macro is.* Don't worry, my friend, I'll teach you. All you need to know now is that, whether you're dealing with menopause symptoms, joint pain, or simply want to feel stronger and more energetic, paying attention to your macros can make a world of difference.

WHAT IS A MACRO, ANYWAY?

Macronutrients are simply protein, carbs, and fats, and *micronutrients* are the nutritional value – vitamins and minerals – found in food. If you get smarter about your balance of protein, carbs, and fats, you can really make a difference to your body shape. This balance allows you to avoid going on a low-calorie diet to lose weight.

On the standard Western or American diet, it's difficult to get this balance right because the standard diet is too low in protein and too high in carbs, and not the complex carbs that I recommend. They tend to be high in refined sugar and white flour.

Conversely, people who are on a ketogenic diet (which I know is very popular) eat plenty of protein and fat, but not many carbohydrates, which, as we've discussed in the previous chapter, is not good for women in perimenopause or menopause. Nevertheless, you need to consume protein in levels much higher than you're used to.

For women over forty, it's important not just to consider calories, but the balance of protein, carbohydrates, and fats. It's got everything to do with your hormones and how they behave. Many experts will tell you all you need to do is simply be in a calorie deficit, and you can lose weight. Well, that's just not true for women over forty. A calorie deficit means burning more energy than you're putting in as fuel. I did this, and it wasn't working. This doesn't mean that you don't consider calories – of course, you still need to be in a calorie deficit, but you also need to consider how you're balancing your hormones. This is time to start looking at your macronutrient intake.

The diet I am about to discuss is much like something you'd find in a bodybuilding style diet. However, it's not all chicken, broccoli, and rice; it has more variety. Rather than just getting your protein sources from chicken, you can get it from fish or beef. Those who are plant-based can get their protein from tofu or beans. Supplementing with protein powder will also increase your protein intake, and you can use protein powder for snacks. Rather than eating a cookie (you tend to have something that's carb-based in the afternoon as a snack or in the morning), you can make protein shake with some berries and protein powder.

Complex carbohydrates release much more slowly in your system, so it's good to look at things like brown rice, potatoes, oatmeal, and whole grains. People aren't afraid of fats anymore because of the popularity of the ketogenic diet, but it's still important to get good fats in and avoid processed fats. What I'm suggesting differs from what's recommended on a ketogenic diet, like processed meats and cheeses. Nuts, nut butters, olive oil, coconut oil, MCT oil, avocados, and oily fish are going to help balance your hormones, and they're great non-inflammatory foods.

I recommend that you start incorporating non-inflammatory foods into your diet. These are just natural foods – they walk, fly, swim, or grow. It's fresh or frozen chicken, fish, or beef that hasn't been processed or prepackaged. Green, leafy vegetables are great because they've got a lot of antioxidants, as do berries and tomatoes.

"Whole" foods are important, and I always recommend whole grains rather than foods with white flour, because white flour has been processed to remove parts of the grain. Additionally, whole grains are less inflammatory – they won't give you an insulin spike. I can't stress this importance enough: most menopausal women will suffer with insulin resistance, so you want to make sure you are avoiding foods that will cause that insulin spike. Whole grains are also good, although for women with thyroid issues or autoimmune diseases, gluten free food is a better option because for women with thyroid issues, gluten and dairy can cause inflammation.

Eggs and dairy are great protein sources. Greek yogurt and kefir (a fermented yogurt) are non-inflammatory; however, people with thyroid issues generally need to avoid dairy. Other non-inflammatory foods, like avocados, oily fish, olive oil, and dark chocolate (70 percent) are all non-inflammatory, have antioxidants, and are great for balancing out hormones.

HOW MANY CALORIES SHOULD YOU CONSUME?

You are often told if you want to lose weight or fat to go really low calorie with your diet. Anything under 1,300 calories a day is generally too low to live on and be able to function properly. When you are consistently low on calories, you actually damage your metabolism. When your calories are extremely low, you get hungry, then binge eat and yo-yo diet. It's much healthier to stick to a higher calorie range and be consistent over time.

This is a hard message to get across to women. Many weight loss experts and doctors often suggest to just take your calories lower, but it doesn't work well in the long term – it just destroys your metabolism. The good news is that metabolism can be fixed. You can boost it with diet and exercise.

The normal calorie range for fat loss in most women is between 1,500 and 2,000 calories a day. Some women, even older women, can lose weight on 2,000 calories a day; they may be over 200 pounds or quite tall. The more you weigh, the more calories you're going to burn.

DOING THE MATH

There are many ways to calculate calories, most of which are too complex to address here, so I've come up with an easy formula. Before I go into that, you can get an accurate understanding of what your maintenance calories are by downloading an app like MyFitnessPal or Cronometer to track everything you're currently eating. If you're staying at the same weight, those are your maintenance calories. You can also go online and use a website like calculator.net, searching "Fitness & Health Calculators" where you can plug in some simple stats like your height, weight, and age to find your maintenance calories. Women who are doing the strength training and cardio that I recommend will need between 1,800 to 2,300 calories for maintenance. Once you've calculated your maintenance calories, subtract between 200 and 300 calories to ensure you are burning more calories than you are consuming. In this instance, you'll need between 1,600 to 2,000 calories a day to lose weight.

You want your calories to be as high as possible and still be able to lose weight because it's going to be more comfortable for you, and it won't slow your metabolism. It's also going to give you a buffer; if you hit a plateau, you can always drop your calories. If you start off too low, there's nowhere to go, and it's not going to work for your metabolism in the long run.

You've worked out how many calories you need to do to lose weight, so now you need to think about your macros.

Like I mentioned earlier, you need to be taking in one gram of protein for every pound in body weight, or if you weigh over 170 pounds, your goal body weight. For many people, that's about 120 to 160 grams of protein. Well, that's a lot of protein, and most people probably find in the standard American diet, they're probably only having something like 70 or 80 grams of protein. So, it's a big change in the way that you're eating.

So, say you've got 150 grams of protein, for argument's sake, let's add your carbs. For most women over forty, you'll need between 100 and 200 grams of carbs. If you've plugged that number into MyFitnessPal or Cronometer (an app similar to MyFitnessPal that I recommend to women), you've plugged your protein intake in and what you've got left is what you can have as carbs and fats. So, we'll be able to have 150 grams of carbs, and then whatever's leftover is fat.

I know I've been talking about grams, and in the US there's a different system, but you're going to have much better accuracy if you're calculating your macros in grams. Roughly speaking, you should be eating 35 to 40 percent protein, 30 to 35 percent carbs, and 30 percent fat per day when you actually start to weigh your food out.

LEVERAGING YOUR MACRO MAKEOVER

Michelle's journey highlights the importance of nutrition and the role of macronutrients in achieving one's health and fitness goals. Her transformation, fueled by a methodical approach to balancing protein, carbohydrates, and fats, underscores the power of dietary adjustments. However, understanding macros is only one piece of the puzzle. To truly revolutionize your body and health, the right exercise regimen is equally crucial.

This brings us to the next vital component of your transformation: strength training. As you'll see in the following chapter, investing in your body's future through strength training can not only enhance your metabolism but also allow you to enjoy a more vibrant and energetic life. Just as Michelle embraced the macro makeover, it's time to delve into the world of sweat equity, where you'll learn how to build muscle, burn fat, and truly redefine your body. Let's explore how combining these nutritional insights with effective strength training can lead to remarkable, sustainable results.

If you would like to learn more, you can go to my website, melissaneill.com/plan.

7

SWEAT EQUITY – INVESTING IN YOUR BODY'S FUTURE

As a nutritionist, Spela knew the importance of a healthy lifestyle, yet her own fitness journey had become a series of starts and stops. Despite her knowledge, something was missing – a crucial piece of the puzzle that kept her from achieving the transformation she desperately wanted.

For years, Spela had battled with perfectionism. If she couldn't follow a diet or exercise plan flawlessly, she would give up entirely. This all-or-nothing mentality had left her feeling defeated and discouraged. "In the past, I would have expected perfection from myself," Spela admitted. This expectation often led to self-sabotage, causing her to abandon her efforts at the first sign of a setback.

Spela's turning point came when she decided to join my challenge. Little did she know that this decision would not only transform her body but also revolutionize her approach to fitness and life.

As Spela delved into the program, she discovered what had been missing all along – a structured training plan. "It was the first time in my life that I had a leg day, upper body day, and things like that," she shared. This revelation was transformative. The clear, easy-to-follow workouts provided the framework she needed to stay consistent and see results.

But the real breakthrough came in Spela's mindset. She realized that "imperfect action is what's important." Instead of letting one slip-up derail her entire journey, Spela learned to get back on track quickly. "Even though I had a few wobbles on the way, I managed to always get back on it and didn't let one day turn into two or three days," she explained.

This shift in perspective was crucial. As I will show you in this chapter, consistency in exercise is key, especially for women over forty. Spela's story perfectly illustrates why the structured approach to strength training that I recommend is so effective. By alternating between upper and lower body workouts, as outlined in the split routine later in the chapter, Spela was able to challenge her muscles consistently without overtraining.

The results of Spela's newfound consistency and structured approach were remarkable. Not only did she see physical changes, but she also experienced a profound mental and psychological transformation. "I feel so much happier now," Spela beamed. "I'm so much more cheerful, have more energy, and of course, that has a positive impact on my relationships with friends and family."

You see, so many women – even industry experts like Spela – get exercise wrong. It's not your fault or their fault. It's not like you decided to put in all that hard work just so you can say, "Well, it was fun doing the *wrong* exercises today!"

Sadly, most women are conditioned into the wrong thinking when it comes to exercise, and I'm going to help you out of it.

WHY STRENGTH TRAINING?

Strength training is going to be the main form of exercise that enables you to increase your metabolism. It's going to enable you to burn fat but also eat more food, which means you can take a bit more pleasure from life by not starving yourself, which is quite a miserable existence.

You shouldn't be afraid of strength training. Women, particularly in their forties, fifties, and beyond, see pictures of female competitive body-builders who are in bigger categories like figure and physique and think, *that's what I'm going to look like if I lift weights.* But you cannot get like that! Competitive bodybuilders have often been training for years in a calorie surplus or take performance enhancing drugs.

I've been strength training for over seven years; it's actually hard to put on significant amounts of muscle unless you've got a propensity toward it. Some women can put on muscle a bit more easily than other women because it's in their genes, but when you get to a certain age, it's actually very hard to do. It takes a lot of work. All you're going to do is get what many describe as "toned." You're not going to get "bulky" – that's a complete myth.

THE SPLIT

The split is the cornerstone of my method for losing weight for women over forty. Beginners can get great results by strength training two or three times a week to get established, but the method that I like to use, and one that is common in the bodybuilding community, is doing an upper and lower body split. What that means is doing your upper body two days a week and your lower body two days a week. This gives your muscles time to recover. You don't want to work the same muscles day after day. Muscle needs time to rest and grow, which is why you should alternate between different muscle groups. For women of a lower weight who don't have so much weight to lose, you're talking about a body recomposition – that doesn't necessarily mean that you're going to lose pounds. What you're going to do is reduce your body fat and put on lean muscle, which can mean that you either stay the same weight or you may see an increase in weight.

Even for larger women, it is a very effective method. A lot of women think, *well, if I weigh more, I need to do cardio to get my weight down,* but you actually need to be doing strength training. It's the same method. Whether you have ten pounds to lose or a hundred pounds to lose, your main focus should be strength training.

If you're a cardio bunny like I was, you need to rethink your workouts and prioritize your strength training. Lifting weights can be done at home or at the gym. However, if you've been lifting at home for a significant amount of time, you'll find you may need to buy new, heavier weights or join a gym because your body gets used to your workouts. The way that you increase your muscle mass is through hypertrophy – the ability to grow muscle – which you can only achieve by consistently challenging the muscle. If you're just lifting the same amount of weight over and over again, for weeks on end, it will not continue to have an impact. You have to keep challenging your muscles.

ACHIEVING HYPERTROPHY

Working out at a gym is more demanding. There, it's easier to push yourself harder. At a gym, you can use heavier weights, whereas at home, you'll be limited to the number of weights you have, unless you're lucky and have a very well-equipped home gym. Working out at home is a challenge because you can't always take a heavier weight when your body adjusts to it. It's always a really good idea whether you're at home or at the gym to just go as heavy as possible for the full benefit of strength training. You shouldn't be afraid to lift heavy.

As women, there is another myth that we've been conditioned to think – that somehow we're going to turn into men and look manly, but that's not true at all. You'll have a feminine, sculpted body by lifting heavy weights and just put the muscle on that you've lost through the aging process. Strength training gives you a better opportunity to burn fat and burn more fat. So, with lifting heavy, what I recommend (and there's a sample workout in this chapter) is the eight to twelve repetition range, which is its optimum for hypertrophy.

Of course, there are other rep ranges; you could do

light weights at twenty reps, but you're not going to get hypertrophy with that. Conversely, you can do heavy weights, with a low rep range, which is going to build your strength. That's something powerlifters do, but it's not going to shape and define your muscles unless it's combined in sets which have high reps and low reps. So, that's why you want to stay in the eight to twelve rep range. The last few reps that you do should feel very challenging and tough to finish – some people even work to failure. Now, you don't have to work to failure, though some trainers will tell you otherwise.

Women always ask me, "How heavy should I be lifting?" There isn't a "one size fits all" answer. It's important that you don't compare yourself to other women and think, *well, they're lifting this amount of weight. That's what I should be lifting.* Everyone is different, so I can't give you specifics on how much weight you should be lifting. It's about how it feels for you.

What you normally find is that women are stronger on their lower bodies, but that's not always the case; some women are blessed with arm strength. If you do certain sports, you're going to have strength in certain areas of your body. If you've done lots of cycling, but you've never done any strength training, your legs are going to be strong, so you can probably lift heavier on your lower body than someone else who is a newcomer.

If you've had more experience lifting, you're going to get better over time and be able to lift heavier. Nevertheless, it's really important to focus on getting the technique right.

You also need to consider how many carbohydrates you're taking in prior to a workout, because more carbohydrates will enable you to lift heavier. That's where the nutrition plan that we talked about helps. Having enough carbohydrates in your system will allow you to be strong enough to perform the strength training exercises, and protein is going to give you protein synthesis after you've worked out.

I see women make this mistake often – either they're not taking in enough food, or they're not actually eating enough carbohydrates to support strength training, so they don't make any progress. They'll tell me, "I'm strength training and nothing's happening. I don't see a difference." Then they'll tell me they're doing keto. Well, the reason they're not seeing a difference is because keto has little to no carbohydrates! It's very difficult to build muscle on keto – you won't find anyone in the competitive bodybuilding community doing keto because it doesn't work as a way of trying to build muscle. It's also very difficult to build muscle when you're over forty, so you need to do everything you can to help your body to grow muscle and that is done just as much by nutrition as the actual training.

Have you ever seen people training hard daily at the gym, but their body never seems to change, and they look continually out of shape? That's because they are not paying attention to nutrition enough.

THE BIG MISCONCEPTION

Women are often conditioned to believe that cardio is going to strip you of body fat. That's not entirely wrong. There is a place for cardio, but you do have to do less of it as you get older to lose fat. This is because too much intense cardio, like long distance running, will result in loss of muscle which you cannot afford to have happen when you are over forty, as you need to build and retain muscle.

I find that when I speak to a lot of women, and what I found in my own experience, is that cardio no longer works as well when you're older. Women will do a ton of cardio and not see the results they want and think, wrongly, *well, I need to increase my cardio exercises, so I'm burning more fat.* But they just end up nowhere and completely exhausted. That's what I did. I took up running and ran for miles training for a half marathon, but I actually gained weight! Lots of cardio is one of the worst strategies for women over forty and where I see most women go wrong when it comes to fat loss.

What you need to do is focus your efforts on strength training. This can sound scary, particularly if you haven't done any kind of strength training before. But lifting weights will help build your metabolism because what muscle does is burn calories, and therefore, fat, even when you are just sitting around doing nothing. This is because it increases your basal metabolic rate, which has decreased with age, as we've explored in other chapters.

ADDING HIIT

I recommend that you supplement strength training with high intensity interval training (HIIT). There are all sorts of different ways of doing this. You can do three times a week for between fifteen and thirty minutes on any piece of cardio equipment, such as a cross trainer or rowing machine. You're going to get more efficient at fat burning with HIIT than you will with steady state cardio, and it won't take long if you're consistent. HIIT involves twenty to thirty seconds of very intense, fast paced exercise at sprint speed, followed by thirty seconds to two minutes of walking pace or rest. It's excellent for improving your aerobic fitness level, and therefore your heart health.

The North American Menopause Society has done a study on HIIT and found it to be more effective than steady state cardio for burning menopausal fat. People also have this misconception that it's not good for menopausal women to do HIIT, but they also found that's not true at all. You can push yourselves harder than you think unless you've got specific mobility problems.

Most people can do strength training in some way, shape, or form, but people with mobility issues or a health problem might be unable to do HIIT. If that's the case, I would recommend that you walk about 7,000-plus steps per day to support the strength training. If you're new to exercise, you can just do ten minutes of walking and build up from there.

There's one more thing that's important, and that's rest. When women find it difficult to lose weight, they'll attempt to work out every day during the week, but this is actually something called overtraining. They're putting their body under way too much stress. Perimenopausal women's bodies are going through stress, and strength training every day will only add to it, so make sure to take two days a week off.

You can do "active" rest on your days off, like walking or yoga, but you shouldn't do strength training or HIIT seven days a week. It's just not good for you. I'm a competitive bodybuilder, and I work out five times a week. I make sure to have two rest days, even if I'm close to a show. When I'm about three weeks away from a competition, I start putting in an extra day of cardio but that's because I've got to get incredibly lean.

People would think that I must work out every day, but it is actually counterproductive. It puts the body under so much stress that it can actually make it more difficult to lose weight, gain muscle, or both. Over training can put you at risk of injury and reduce your immune system so you get sick a lot.

WALKING

I absolutely *love* walking as a form of exercise for women over forty. It's so important to keep your body moving and you will burn more calories by simply walking.

Personally, I used to think of walking as the poor cousin of running until I discovered how running was actually preventing me from getting in shape.

Now I love walking. I get out and walk most mornings because there are *huge* physical and mental health benefits.

Not only are you simply going to burn more calories if you incorporate walking, but you are also going to enjoy better health. There have been countless studies that show by implementing walking you are going to reduce your risk of many modern-day diseases.

In the Western world, we are far too sedentary.

This has a damaging effect on our health. You can suffer from musculoskeletal problems by sitting too much and even your digestion can suffer.

Getting outside in particular is really great for your mental health and getting some sunlight on you early in the morning is even more beneficial if you can do it. If you can walk outside in nature, you are going to improve your mood – something that can be really low at the time around menopause.

If you don't walk already, you don't have to make it onerous. You can start with ten minutes a day and build up from there. Ideally, you want to average at least 7,000 steps per day which works out at around three miles.

If you live somewhere extremely hot or cold, you can use a treadmill but do swap that for outdoor walks at the times of year when the weather is not so extreme.

SAMPLE HOME WORKOUT PLAN

To balance out all your changing body's needs, here is a sample exercise plan you can follow.

You can find workouts like these by going to the app store or Google Play and downloading my Body By Bikini app which has a *free* 7 day program with follow-along videos. Go to melissaneill.com/plan to download.

This is a home workout plan, but you can find a gym alternative in my app.

Days	Strength	Suggested HIIT Cardio Days
Day 1	Workout 1 (Legs)	Rest
Day 2	Workout 2 (Upper Body)	15-30 minutes HIIT
Day 3	Rest	Rest
Day 4	Workout 4 (Glutes and Legs)	15-30 minutes HIIT
Day 5	Rest	Optional 15-30 minutes HIIT
Day 6	Workout 5 (Upper Body)	15-30 minutes HIIT
Day 7	Rest	Rest

Please warm up before each strength training session with some of the following exercises without weight:

- Glute bridges
- Glute kickbacks on floor
- Squats
- Push-ups
- Lunges
- Cat-cow

Then cool down at the end with some stretches.

Day 1: Legs

1. 3 to 5 sets of 8 to 12 squats (dumbbells on shoulders)
2. 3 sets of 10 on each leg reverse lunges dumbbells hands by side
3. 3 sets of 10 each leg Bulgarian split squats (1 foot behind you on bench)
4. 3 to 5 sets of 8 to 12 dumbbell hip thrusts (shoulders supported on your bench) or glute bridges (lying on floor)
5. 3 sets of 10 to 12 stiff leg deadlift

Day 2: Upper body

1. 3 sets of 8 to 10 triceps dips on bench
2. Dumbbell overhead press 3 sets of 10
3. Dumbbell supersets of 10 each of: Lateral raises, front raises
4. 3 sets of 10 to 15 dumbbell bicep curls
5. 3 sets of 10 push ups
6. 3 sets of 10 Arnold press (start with hands facing towards you then press up over your head and turn hands to face away)

Day 3: Rest

Day 4: Glute-focused leg day

1. 3 to 5 sets of 8 to 12 sumo squats with dumbbells
2. 3 sets of 10 to 12 Romanian deadlifts
3. 3 sets of 10 on each leg dumbbell step-ups - use a bench or chair
4. 5 sets of 15 to 20 hip thrusts or glute bridges with dumbbell
5. 4 sets of 10 fire hydrants with glute band

Day 5: Rest or active rest (like walking)

Day 6: Upper body

1. 3 sets of 10 overhead press with dumbbells
2. 4 sets of 30 second plank
3. 3 sets of 8 to 10 dips on bench or chair
4. 4 sets of 10 dumbbell bent over row with dumbbells
5. 3 sets of 10 bicep curls
6. 3 sets of 10 dumbbell lateral raises superset with front raises

Day 7: Rest

THE BALANCE OF EFFORT AND RECOVERY

As we've seen, incorporating strength training into your fitness routine is crucial for increasing metabolism, burning fat, and enjoying a more dynamic and fulfilling life. However, as you embark on this journey of physical transformation, it's essential to recognize that pushing your body to its limits must be balanced with adequate rest and recovery. Without this balance, you risk overtraining and compromising your progress, health, and well-being.

Strength training and HIIT are powerful tools for reshaping your body, but they can also be taxing, especially for women over forty. This is where the importance of rest and recovery comes in. As we move into the next chapter, we'll delve into why rest is just as crucial as your workouts. We'll explore strategies to ensure you're giving your body the time it needs to repair, rejuvenate, and build muscle effectively.

In the next chapter, you'll meet Tracy, whose story illustrates the vital role of rest in achieving and maintaining fitness goals. Her journey highlights how balancing effort with rest can lead to sustainable success. Let's explore the often-overlooked aspect of fitness: the power of proper rest and recovery.

If you would like video tutorials of the workouts

described in this chapter, go to melissaneill.com/plan and download my *free* 7-day program.

8

DREAM BIG, REST WELL

For years, Tracy put everyone else's needs before her own, leaving her depleted and disconnected from herself. The idea of embarking on a fitness journey seemed daunting, almost impossible. How could she find the energy to transform her body when she could barely make it through the day?

But deep down, Tracy knew something had to change. She yearned to prove to herself that she could accomplish something solely for her own benefit. When she discovered my challenge, Tracy saw it as her chance to reclaim her health and vitality.

From the start, Tracy approached the challenge with unwavering determination. She committed to following the meal plan and workout routine to the letter, allowing herself only one small deviation – a single salad – throughout the entire program. This level of dedication was admirable, but as I often caution in this chapter, it's crucial to balance intense effort with proper rest and recovery.

As Tracy progressed through the challenge, she began to understand the delicate balance between pushing herself and allowing time for rest. The final three weeks proved to be particularly grueling, testing her resolve both emotionally and mentally. "I had a lack of energy, a lack of motivation," Tracy admitted. Yet, she persevered, recognizing that these moments of fatigue were not signs of weakness, but signals from her body that rest was needed.

Listen, if you're a woman over forty, like me and like Tracy, then I know you're not getting enough sleep. How? Because women over forty are almost always superheroes. They're moms, friends, spouses, caregivers, employees, bosses, and more. And Tracy's story is a great example of that. Her story proves that adequate rest is crucial for muscle recovery, hormone balance, and overall well-being. Tracy's moments of low energy and motivation were likely her body's way of signaling the need for more recovery time.

Despite the challenges, Tracy pushed through, completing every workout and sticking to her nutrition plan. However, her journey highlights the need for a balanced approach. While dedication is admirable, it's equally important to listen to your body and allow for adequate rest. And that's what I want to talk about in this chapter: sleep and rest, one of the cornerstones of weight loss and healthy living. As a woman over forty, you've got to look after your long-term health and your hormone health – getting enough sleep and rest are essential to this.

DIFFERENT ASPECTS OF REST

Let's talk about getting enough rest between training sessions. You need at least two days off a week to ensure that your body has rested adequately between training sessions. When you don't see progress, the knee jerk reaction is to increase your activity; you might start working out strenuously seven days a week. But this will hinder your progress.

As I've discussed in earlier chapters, the way that you're going to lose weight is by building your metabolism through strength training; your muscles develop when you're resting. So, if you're not resting enough, your muscles won't grow or develop, and that means that you're not going to increase your metabolism or burn fat. It is, therefore, important to have clear rest days and not train the same muscles on consecutive days.

When you look at my suggested training programs, you'll see that if you do a leg day or a lower body day, you do an upper body day the next day – you're not working the same muscles on consecutive days. On rest days, we can do active *rest*, like walking and yoga. As older women, we generally need more rest than we did when we were younger. We do not need to train day after day. I find that I need more recovery time to perform better in the gym than I did ten or twenty years ago. I also take a rest week three or four times per year. I used to fear rest week. In other words, this would be a vacation where there wasn't a gym so I would take my own resistance bands and skipping rope to work out. Now, I use some of my vacations as a chance to recover. There's nothing wrong with taking equipment with you, but if you haven't had a rest week in say twelve weeks, you can use your break as a chance to recover.

This brings me to overtraining, which is not only training seven days a week, but also doing too much training. You don't need to go into the gym and do two and a half hour sessions. Overtraining can cause a lot of damage to your body, because, unless you're a professional athlete, your body is not equipped to do that amount of training. Your immune system really takes a nosedive when overtraining, and that can cause you to get sick.

You may also end up with injuries because your body hasn't had time to recover.

MY OVERTRAINING STORY

I've learned about how damaging overtraining can be. As you know, I am a bikini competitor. The two or three weeks leading up to the show are intense. There is something called peak week, which is the week before the show. In essence, I go to the gym for two and a half hours per session (which I wouldn't recommend you do under any circumstances unless you're getting ready for stage like me!).

For example, I was doing about an hour and fifteen minutes of strength training and an hour and fifteen to an hour and thirty minutes of cardio. It is intense cardio as well, like running up the stair climber with a weighted vest. This type of strenuous exercise helps drop that extra body fat the week before the show. At the same time, during peak week, your calories are lower than what you're used to – about 1,500 calories. Because you're burning so many calories during training, your deficit is going to be quite big.

It's really grueling and punishing on the body. On some days, you're almost reduced to tears; you get emotional because you're pushing yourself to the limit mentally and physically to get through it. It's really not for the faint of heart.

In 2021, I did two shows back-to-back. I had done this when I was fifty-two years old no problem. But this time, at fifty-four years old, the following week after the shows, I booked a photography shoot. I did two peak weeks, which were incredibly grueling, and then I did a *third* peak week.

In hindsight, I really didn't need to do the third week because all I needed to do was maintain the body that I had achieved for the two shows to prepare for the photo shoot. I should have dropped the extreme train-ing; I should have just done my strength training sessions and eaten sensibly. When you've achieved your goal body, it's quite easy to maintain what you have got through a maintenance training and diet protocol that doesn't need to be extreme.

Two days before the photography shoot, I got sick with a virus. Thankfully, it wasn't COVID, but it took me about two weeks to recover. I then went to Croatia on vacation. During the second week, while I was recovering from the first virus in Croatia, I tested posi-tive for COVID. I didn't have any symptoms at first, but then I came down with quite severe symptoms, even though I have been double vaccinated.

This was a classic case of overtraining. My immune system had just basically taken a nosedive. I haven't competed again since then. And if I don't feel ready, I won't even compete for a few years.

This experience taught me a valuable lesson that the menopausal body is not as resilient as a young woman's body. I also learned how vital it is that you pay attention to and listen to your body. If something feels off, don't push through; take rest.

AGING AND INJURIES

As you get older, you're going to be more prone to injuries, pain, and muscular or joint problems – this is even experienced by top athletes. Your approach to fitness and exercise should be positive, but you must understand that your body has limitations.

In exercise, there's *good* pain and *bad* pain. Good pain is muscle soreness – it means that you're growing your muscles. Some people experience extreme muscle soreness when they start strength training. This is normal and you can use Epsom bath salts, branched chain amino acids (an amino acid found in protein that helps with protein synthesis and muscle recovery), or do a lot of stretching to overcome it.

The bad pain is from painful joints. Back pain is also common in the Western world, as is knee, shoulder, and hip pain. If you're experiencing any of these, you need to stop working out that part of your body temporarily, and when you do work out, know the limits of what your body can handle. My maximum one repetition squat is about 200 pounds; I know that if I attempt to go over that, I'm going to feel pain in my back. So, I never lift over that weight because I listen to my body. On some days, I may not be able to get anywhere near that kind of weight, especially if I am in a calorie deficit. If you have pain in your joints, you should stop exercising immediately. If you've got any ongoing issues, and you know your own body, you have to work around those. For example:

- If you've got bad knees, doing exercises with high-impact movements won't be appropriate. So, you need to modify the moves to make them low impact.
- When at the gym, don't max out on heavy weights that you know are going to cause problems. Make the weight a little challenging but still comfortable.
- If you've got knee problems and lunges are difficult, you can try lunges without weight or do glute kickbacks instead.

- You will reach a plateau on the weight you can lift, so instead, use other techniques like slowing the movement down – count for two to three seconds – and you will really find this challenging.
- Do *supersets* – when one exercise is performed straight after the other. You won't want to go heavier on those exercises because you're performing one set, moving on to a different exercise, and performing another set on that exercise. This really avoids the need for going to your maximum weight capacity.
- You can also drop sets, where you start off on your heaviest weight for ten repetitions in the first set. Then, without a rest, you drop the weight down to half and do ten more reps. This will also help you avoid the need to increase the weight because you're going to hit a plateau with how heavy you can lift.

These techniques are great for people who are lifting at an intermediate and advanced level, particularly in an older age group because you just can't keep loading up the bar with more and more weight. They also allow you to achieve something called *progressive overload,* which is a continued challenge to your muscle. That's what you want to achieve, but you're protecting your joints at the same time.

AVOIDING ILLNESS

When I'm traveling a lot, and I'm dehydrated, if I try to go to the gym in that condition, I just don't get a good workout. I can't lift as well as I normally do. If you feel "off," or you're tired, you're probably not going to have a good training session. As with joint pain, that's the day it's likely that you're going to have an injury. It may be a good day to rest instead. I'm a big proponent of doing what I've been talking about in this book and doing it consistently over time. Taking a day's rest in the whole scheme of things is not going to be a deal breaker, because you're being consistent over time.

Rest days are as important as your workouts, because too much training can make you ill and cause injuries. As you remember, I overtrained because I prepared for two shows and a photoshoot and made myself sick. I believe it's because my immune system was really low, and I learned my lesson. I've since pulled back my schedule. I tend to do strength training four times a week, and I do one HIIT session once a week. That's pretty much all I do. Depending on the time of year and what's coming up in my schedule, I might put in some cardio activity, but I won't do more than thirty minutes.

If you've got a virus, the worst thing you can do is train through it – you have to let your body rest, and you've got to feed your body properly. When you're sick it isn't the time to be cutting back on food. Go for nutritious foods – eat lots of fresh fruits and vegetables. Feed your body to restore it and only go back when you're feeling well enough. If you're getting a lot of viruses, do have a look at your training you might want to pull it back because it's just not going to be good for you in the long term, and it won't be good for weight loss anyway.

MUSCLE GROUPS AND REST

When you work out with weights, you may pick up an injury. It's important to seek professional help, even if it's a low-level injury.

A woman who was on my Lean and Strong program contacted me and told me she had tennis elbow and asked if I had any modifications. Luckily, she lives near me, and I told her I didn't think she could train, but I knew a good physiotherapist who turned my life around, and I gave her his details.

That's exactly what I would recommend you do if you've got an injury that's preventing you from working out. In the long-term, seeing a professional is going to help you get back on track a bit more quickly from that injury. Don't return to exercise until that professional tells you it's okay to do so.

I get a lot of people messaging me on social media asking me what they would do in the event of an injury, but I'm not the right person to speak to about that. I train people to exercise and help them with nutrition. I'm not a medical professional and what you need is a physiotherapist or sports massage therapist who can give you rehabilitation exercises. It's important to stick to these diligently and only go back to the gym when the medical professional says you can. You may have to avoid some exercises initially, but you can start doing exercises that you know are safe, or that your physiotherapist or your doctor approved.

Often, a physiotherapist will say it's okay to swim and this can be really good for joints. You could return to walking as well. In fact, walking is probably the easiest thing for you to start with, then you can gradually build up from there.

In short, always listen to your body and don't be afraid that you've lost progress because it will come back. People worry when they've had a long time away from exercise due to sickness or injury. They think it's going to be difficult coming back, but you haven't lost all your progress. It takes a long time to lose muscle. Even when I spent six weeks away, I didn't really lose muscle.

Just take care that when you are returning to the gym, you're doing so at the right time, and that you've sought the proper medical advice to help you return.

SLEEP AND MENOPAUSE

Making sure you take rest days in the week and avoid overtraining isn't the only way to improve your overall rest. Sleep, especially for women over forty, is also crucial. Sleep used to be underplayed in the fitness industry, but it plays a vital role in weight loss. However, when you're in perimenopause or menopause, it's really difficult to get sleep. I know, because I too have difficulty sleeping. So, I'm going to talk about the reasons why sleep is so important and give you some strategies that you can use to try and improve your sleep.

Often times when you're going through peri-menopause and menopause you are not getting enough high-quality sleep because you're not going to bed early enough, then you're getting up too early, or you're just getting broken sleep. This can cause your metabolism to slow and can cause glucose intolerance and insulin resistance.

The deep sleep you get builds bone and muscle, repairs and regenerates tissues, and strengthens your immune system. To get this high-quality deep sleep, you should be sleeping according to the circadian rhythm, which is your body's internal clock. The optimum cycle for your body is to go to bed early and get up early at the same time every day.

You know, if you have a really poor night's sleep, you are more likely to get cravings; you may tend to overeat the day after. Studies have shown that a lack of sleep impacts your neurotransmitters. Hormones called ghrelin and leptin, which are really important for appetite control, go off and this results in serious cravings especially for high-fat, high-sugar foods.

Sleep really does impact your body's ability to lose weight and will affect your overall general health. If you can get a good night's sleep, you are going to have much more success with weight loss. It's likely that your sleep pattern has become irregular since peri-menopause or even before. And, in fact, that is often the first signal you get that you're approaching peri-menopause – you keep waking up at night.

I wake up most nights because I have to get up to go to the bathroom, which is also common for women our age. Some nights are better than others, but some nights, once you wake up, it can be difficult to get back to sleep. I also experienced extreme night sweats and was waking up six times in the night with my night clothes and sheets soaked. I started taking hormone replacement therapy (HRT) in the form of estrogen and proges-terone. This has been totally transformative for me and enabled me to get a good night's sleep. Not everyone will want to go down the route of HRT, but if you are struggling with symptoms and you have done everything I have recommended in this book to adjust your lifestyle and you are still getting symptoms like I did, then HRT is definitely worth a discussion with your doctor.

There are some strategies you can employ to improve your sleep, and since I implemented them myself, I've found that my sleep quality has improved, and I feel much better.

WHAT TO DO TO IMPROVE YOUR SLEEP

Here are some tips to make yourself more conducive to sleep:

- Avoid tech in your bedroom. While it is hard, you should discipline yourself and avoid looking at your phone or computer for at least an hour before bed. Devices give off blue light that's really stimulating. Even if you find it easy to fall asleep, using tech before bed can cause you to wake up later in the night.

- Keep your bedroom free of clutter, which actually causes all kinds of stress. Make your bedroom a cozy and comfortable place to be.

- Try supplements. I've fallen into a pattern of waking up every night and then not being able to go back to sleep. I started using a supplement called ashwagandha, and I find it helpful. Don't rely on this supplement night after night, but just use them to help you get back into the pattern of sleeping again. You can also try melatonin or CBD oil.

- Try listening to something relaxing. Relaxing audio to promote mindfulness can be found on YouTube or any app store, and these can be helpful before you go to sleep, as long as you're not looking at a screen while you're doing it.

- Keep your bedroom cool with a window open, a fan, or air conditioning. You will find you can easily get too hot at this stage

in life and the goal is to keep cool, which
will improve your sleep quality.

- Finally, it depends on where you live (e.g.,
  how hot it is and what time of year), but a
  weighted blanket is also helpful. Many
  people find them very relaxing.

In the next chapter, I'm going to talk about stress,
because it can also influence your weight significantly.

9

KEEP CALM AND LOSE WEIGHT

When someone joins my program, one of the first things we do is have the client take "before" photos. It's a scary task, but it's necessary. In order to solve a problem, you need to be able to assess a situation accurately.

After participating in one of my weight loss challenges, I asked Juanita how it was going. She had just recently downloaded the "before" photos she took at the beginning of the challenge, bringing back all of those old feelings.

"Looking at the first picture I took," she said, "I can see the old me in the sense of lacking confidence, lacking self-esteem, fearful, just not happy, doubtful – all these emotions existed internally, but I didn't realize how much it showed on the outside. I didn't even have the confidence to wear a bikini."

Like many women in midlife, Juanita found herself balancing the demands of work, family, and personal well-being. The stress of juggling multiple responsibilities had taken its toll, not just on her body, but also on her mind and spirit. Yikes.

"Every single day was a battle," Juanita recalled of the beginning days of the weight loss challenge. "Every single day I had to keep focused. Every single day I had to tell myself it can be done, and I had to be determined and keep on."

This daily mental workout became the cornerstone of Juanita's transformation. As I will discuss in this chapter, managing stress is crucial for women over forty, particularly for those going through perimenopause or menopause. Juanita's approach of consciously reframing her thoughts and staying focused aligned perfectly with the stress management strategies I recommend.

As Juanita strengthened her "mental muscle," she noticed changes not just in her mindset, but in her physical appearance. The connection between mental well-being and physical health, which I emphasize throughout this book, became evident in Juanita's journey. She was becoming stronger, a force to be reckoned with.

One of the most significant changes for Juanita was her newfound confidence. The woman who once shied away from wearing a bikini now felt comfortable and confident in her skin. This shift in self-perception is a powerful example of how managing stress and improving mental well-being can positively impact body image and overall happiness.

And as Juanita became more organized and disciplined, she found herself happier. This inner joy was reflected in her smile – a change she noticed immediately when comparing her before and after photos. You see, that's the thing about your inner world – it will always show on your face, no matter how hard you think you hide it. So, what's the alternative?

Easy. Well, kind of...Put in the hard work to manage the stress properly, to find happiness again, and it will show proudly.

The impact of Juanita's transformation rippled out to her family life as well. As I often tell my clients, when we take care of ourselves and manage our stress effectively, we're better equipped to nurture our relationships. Juanita found that her improved self-esteem and reduced stress levels led to better relationships with her family members.

Women over forty are particularly susceptible to the negative effects of stress on our hormones and weight loss efforts. By focusing on her mental well-being, Juanita was able to create a positive cycle:

reduced stress led to better physical results, which in turn further reduced her stress levels.

In the Western world, we lead very busy, stressful lives, and there's a big connection between stress and weight loss. This becomes even more apparent when you get into middle age around menopause.

I work with a lot of women in the United States, and I believe that their lives are particularly stressful compared to other parts of the world, with the societal pressure to work harder and make more money. I think a great deal of value is placed on financial status rather than quality of life.

In middle age, you're working full time. You're often running a household and taking care of the bills as well. You're doing everything. Often, you've got this "sandwich" situation, where you have kids or teenagers in addition to elderly parents. The pandemic increased the stress on people's lives even more, because you spent more time at home working or home schooling. During that time, some people were also laid off and now that you're back to work, inflation has caused the price of everything to go up. These are very stressful events, and they all occurred within a short period of time.

WHY STRESS MATTERS MORE AS WE AGE

As I've discussed, as you age, you're going to have lower levels of hormones. So, when you're in perimenopause or menopause, your hormones are going to be out of balance.

Stress changes your hormone levels – specifically cortisol, triiodothyronine (T_3), and thyroxine (T_4) in your thyroid function, and also insulin. Stress is going to make changes to those hormones and impacts your body's ability to lose weight. You're going to be more prone to storing fat. It's important that you not only look at how much you're eating, but also your stress levels and how much rest you are getting.

Stress can also lead to overeating. Researchers have discovered that you are prone to eating high sugar, high fat, and high salt when you're stressed. The kicker is that if you're highly stressed, it will make weight loss much more difficult, since stress in general is actually a massive contributing factor to weight gain. The reason that stress is a problem is it can cause raised cortisol levels. This in turn can lead to other changes in our sex hormones, like progesterone and testosterone, and these hormones can end up being really out of whack.

Stress can also increase insulin resistance, and insulin resistance plays a big role in why we have gained belly fat. Insulin resistance occurs when our pancreas cannot control our blood sugar levels. It is so common for women over forty, as well as in the Western world at large, that we can almost assume that we are insulin resistant. This can also lead to lots of inflammation in our bodies, and when we've got inflammation, it makes it really difficult to lose weight. In fact, it will lead to the opposite – gaining more weight. So, all in all, if you're stressed, your body is simply going to store more fat.

As women over forty, it's important that you put some strategies in place to help you deal with the stress levels, so that you have a better opportunity for weight loss and storing less fat.

HOW TO REDUCE STRESS IN YOUR LIFE

It's difficult to tell someone who is stressed that they need to reduce their stress levels because it's such a complex thing. One of the things that you need to do is take back control. Sometimes at this stage in life you can feel that you're not in control; you feel controlled by your bosses and your families, and you don't have the control over your own life to make yourself a priority.

It's important that you make yourself a priority. I think when it comes to asking for help as women, you tend to do a lot of the work, but you don't delegate or get support. In the home, much of the work is carried out by women, but you also go out to work. As bread-winners, women tend to do a lot of things to support the family that men as breadwinners just aren't expected to do. When it comes to caring for elderly parents, the responsibility falls on you.

Women tell me that sometimes they're their own worst enemy. They say that they will do the work, even though their husbands, partners, and family members want to give them help. Sometimes you've just got to let go if you want to reduce your stress levels but also find time to work on your health.

I've done it with my own partner I didn't want to release some of those responsibilities onto him. It's hard when you've been doing everything for a long time to ask someone else to chip in, whether it's with cooking, shopping, or helping with the kids. It's good to just let go if you are lucky enough to have help and delegate tasks to family members, particularly if you're someone who works full time and looks after other people.

After releasing that workload, it's about reassessing aspects of your life. In my own life, I looked at what's important and what could be put to one side. Take a look at your responsibilities, whether it's in the home or at work, and release the toxic people in your life. They can bring you down and, by doing so, cause an immense amount of stress.

I did this in my own life because I had a long career in public relations, but I actually wanted to work in fitness and weight loss. Midlife is a great time to reassess everything that you're doing because unhappiness also causes stress if you're doing something that you don't enjoy. Yes, you've got to pay the bills, but now's the time to look at yourself and make some changes. It's never too late.

Even though we may be more financially independent, we can still find that we have financial pressures at this stage in life, adding to our stress. Maybe your kids are going off to college and you are facing university or college fees. Perhaps you had kids young, and your oldest ones are getting married, or perhaps you went back to school to get a degree you always wanted but couldn't when your children were young. Maybe you are divorced, and as a single parent, feel the weight of bills on your own. Aging also brings with it medical conditions, so maybe you are paying for healthcare or medical bills. You may find that you're experiencing other big life-changing events like bereavement, moving house, or divorce. In my middle-aged years, I had to cope with marriage breakdown and divorce, which was really traumatic. At the time, I underestimated what impact this had on my health. Now

looking back, I think, *no wonder I couldn't get in shape.*
My hormones were all over the place and I was under
immense pressure.

With all this pressure and stress, many women find
they actually suffer not just from anxiety and stress,
but also from depression. Often, doctors diagnose their
symptoms incorrectly. Doctors assume that women
need to take antidepressants when actually hormone
replacement therapy can make a massive difference.

Elevated stress levels or depression might mean
that you need to get some outside help – perhaps
through therapy or coaching – because if you're having
difficulties in your life, you often don't feel good about
yourself. Your appearance is changing. Let's face it,
you're aging, and as a woman, you often fear that you're
not worthy anymore. Therapy, counseling, or even
hypnosis can help you to change some things about
your life, including your attitudes. It can show you how
to release some things that are unhelpful and keep the
things that work for you.

You can also have stress that is related to hormones.
Hormone replacement therapy can help with that, but
when it comes to general stress, you've got to work at
reducing it. Coaching, relaxation techniques, taking
time for yourself, and finding something you enjoy can
help you reduce your stress levels.

When I was newly divorced, I realized I'd spent

much of my motherhood putting everybody's needs above my own, and I decided that wasn't going to continue. I was going to do more things that would please myself. Gradually, I started to enjoy life a little bit more. That meant going to music festivals, getting fit in the gym, taking daily walks in the sunshine to boost my mood, taking part in bodybuilding shows, and getting out and about and meeting people. If someone invited me to an event, instead of making excuses, I generally said "yes" a lot more and overtime, I noticed a real difference in my stress levels.

To this day, I relieve stress by dancing. I find it really fun and relaxing. I go out to lots of music events and festivals, and dancing there helps me let my hair down and enjoy myself. But you need to find what you love and do more of it. Make a conscious effort to do the things you love.

Reducing your stress is about finding out what you enjoy, reconnecting with those things, and making time and space for them.

I touched on this briefly here, but in the next chapter, all about mindset, I'm going to talk about how you can start to feel good about yourself because the aging process can take a toll.

10

THE COMEBACK QUEEN – THE MINDSET SHIFT

Stephanie winced as she took her first steps of the day. The familiar ache in her feet, legs, and knees had become her unwelcome morning companion. At 180.7 pounds, with a 32.5-inch waist, Stephanie felt trapped in a body that seemed to be working against her. Shopping for clothes had become an exercise in frustration and self-consciousness.

Determined to reclaim her health and confidence, Stephanie joined my program. Her initial "whys" were straightforward: she wanted to be pain-free and able to walk into any store and buy clothes without feeling insecure. Who wouldn't want that? Especially as a woman over forty.

As Stephanie dove into the program, her body responded. The pounds started to melt away, and her

waist began to shrink. By the end of the 8-week challenge, she had lost an impressive 18.4 pounds, bringing
her weight down to 162.3 pounds. Even more remark-
ably, she had shed 8 inches from her waist, now
measuring 29.5 inches.

But the numbers on the scale and tape measure
were just the beginning of Stephanie's transformation.
As her body changed, so did her focus. She found
herself less concerned with future outcomes and more
excited about present achievements. "I went from
thinking, *what can I have in the future?* to Oh, *I
wonder how many jump squats I can do in a row
without stopping*," Stephanie shared. Her newfound
enthusiasm for push-ups and progressive weightlifting
reflected a profound shift in her approach to fitness.

Stephanie's focus on what she could do in the
present moment, rather than fixating on future goals,
allowed her to tune into her body's capabilities and
challenges. It's the core advice that I can share with
anyone dealing with pain who wants to be healthier:
you must listen to your body and adapt exercises to
your individual needs. But more on that in a second.

Around the third or fourth week of the program,
Stephanie experienced what she described as a
"mindset shift." This transformation in thinking was
perhaps the most significant change of all. "I had a
mindset shift," Stephanie explained. "And that

mindset shift was no longer being a victim of menopause but being a fit, resilient, strong person who can kick menopause in the teeth."

Instead of pushing through pain or ignoring her body's signals, Stephanie learned to challenge herself in ways that were appropriate for her current fitness level. This approach not only led to physical improvements but also helped alleviate the pain that had been plaguing her.

And let's talk about her shift from feeling like a victim of menopause to feeling strong and resilient. I mean really, what a powerful reminder that our mindset plays a crucial role in our fitness journey. This mental strength allowed her to push through challenges and continuously progress in her workouts. It's a secret elixir that anyone can use to power through. Sadly, it's an elixir you can only get if you stay dedicated and committed, just like Stephanie did.

WILL YOU LET AGE DEFINE YOU?

I believe – from my own experience and from working with lots of women – that exercise isn't about putting a barrier up just because you're a certain age. Remember Ernestine Shepherd? Now at eighty-eight, she was at one time the world's oldest female bodybuilder. She's been a fantastic inspiration to me, and I wouldn't be lifting weights if it wasn't for her. If you said to someone twenty or thirty years ago, "You're going to be lifting weights at eighty-eight," they would likely respond with, "It's not safe!" Of course, we've learned over the decades that it is completely safe. You've got to get away from thinking about what is "age appropriate" and don't put boundaries up around certain physical activities.

However, you do need to take care of your health and body when you get to a certain age. Certain activities you take part in may take longer to get better at, and you've got to protect your joints. Nevertheless, you can still learn new things when you're older. For example, I learned to do a pistol squat, pull up, and push-ups in my late forties. I learned to do full, unassisted dips at fifty-two, exercises I had never been able to achieve previously. I just kept chipping away at it, little by little, and got better at it.

MIND OVER MATTER

Mindset is the most important aspect of transforming your body, and the diet and the fitness industry don't talk about this enough. And here's the kicker: mindset is the number one reason most people fail to implement the steps I just taught you. Why? Because it's the hardest thing to change about yourself, and the harder a task is, the more you'll push it off. Not because you're a bad person, but because you are a normal human being. We all do it.

In fact, whenever I post content on how to improve your mindset on YouTube or social media, it more often than not gets ignored. People are looking for quick, easy solutions to how to get in shape, but the fact of the matter is that how I got in shape was 90 percent to do with getting myself in a very different mindset. After all, the mindset I had when I was out of shape wasn't going to be the one to get me back in shape.

Your approach to getting in shape is going to be impacted by what you tell yourself. So, consider this, what is the narrative going on in your head? If it's something like, *I can't do this because it's too difficult,* then you're going to have a rough road ahead. I see a lot of women saying this on social media – they give up before they've even started. They say things like, "I can't meal prep because I have to cook for my kids," "I am too busy to work out," or "I don't have the discipline to eat well." Those are all excuses and ways of putting up a barrier to achieving the body of your dreams. If you want it badly enough and believe in yourself enough, you can succeed. If you're telling yourself you can't do something, it will make it that much harder to actually achieve.

If you stick to your old habits while attempting the

plans in this book, you're going to stay in the same position that you've always been in and never make your transformation. Doing the same things that you did in the past – whether it's with old habits, how you eat, or how you work out – will yield the same results. You need to form new, healthy habits and let go of what you used to do and how you used to think in order to make a real transformation.

The transformation needs to take place in your mind, well before the transformation in your body. I want you to read everything in this chapter, understand the content, take and implement what I am saying. This final piece in the jigsaw puzzle will really be the game changer and make the difference to whether you will succeed or not.

So, as you are implementing this process at home and you run into a setback – whether that's missing a workout day, overeating, or maybe something as (seemingly) simple as negative self-talk, I want you to re-read this chapter. Again. And again. *And again.* Read it however many times it takes to get you back on the horse.

FIND YOUR STRONG REASON WHY

Finding your strong reason why is a very powerful part of the transformation process. It's going to be the foundation that you build everything on. It isn't about goal setting. It's about finding your reason why you are going to get up every morning and train and why you are going to stick to eating the foods that will help you reach your goals and nourish your body.

When I initially went on this journey, my strong reason why was to get through the day. My mental health had taken a dive due to my marriage breaking down, and I literally found it difficult to function. Exercise gave me an opportunity to feel better during the time I was working out and forget about my troubles. Then, as time went on, I wanted to sculpt my body and had a clear idea in my mind's eye that I wanted to get the body of a muscular fitness model. And of course, my ultimate strong reason why was to get on stage and strut around in a sparkly bikini. And now as I'm getting older, I am looking towards old age. I want to live a vibrant life, free from disease, and have the freedom to live a rich and fulfilling life.

You have to find your own strong reason why. It might be for appearance and there is nothing wrong with wanting to look better as looking better will help you feel better. It might be for health. Maybe you want to prevent health issues, or maybe you have some existing health issues that you want to address. As you get older, you're more at risk of heart disease, type 2 diabetes and dementia. The plan I have outlined for you is going to help you prevent those.

Maybe your reason why is an improved quality of life. Maybe you're starting to experience mobility issues like hip, knee, and other joint problems. Maybe you simply lack energy and you're feeling low, and you want the freedom to do the things you want to do without these physical limitations holding you back.

MAKING YOURSELF A PRIORITY

Having an awareness of these habits is key to changing them. Some examples of behaviors that can keep you from reaching your goals are eating too much of the wrong foods, not exercising enough, or not exercising properly. One of the biggest bad habits that women fall into (and that could be a book on its own) is stress eating. If you have these behaviors, you need to let them go to make room for positive habits.

When you're attempting to break old habits and create new ones, the first step is taking responsibility for your actions. I talk to and communicate with women online on an almost daily basis, and I often hear them blame situations for where they are now. For example, they often say, "I got out of shape because of the pandemic." They haven't actually had COVID, but they blame the event because they haven't been able to do the activities that they would normally do, and it's led to their overeating. Another common problem is blaming others for why you are overeating; perhaps you cook for your family, or you go to family get togethers where there is lots of food. However, you are the one who is in control of what goes in your mouth. No one is force feeding you, and you have to accept responsibility for your actions. If you are over-weight (like I was) or obese you have to accept that you are responsible.

In my case, I drank too much alcohol and that was one of the reasons I was stuck and couldn't lose weight. In my younger days, I got away with it, but once I hit my forties, I could no longer do so. I realized that alcohol was holding me back from reaching my goals, so I stopped drinking in the home. I haven't counted but I can only imagine how many calories I reduced taking in just by taking this one action. Then, when I gave up drinking all together, it was like a weight was lifted off me. I no longer had to think about or have a strategy for alcohol. It's one of the best decisions I made in my entire life. It involved a really big leap around my mindset to do that, but I wouldn't be writing this book or making a living from fitness and weight loss if I hadn't shifted my thinking.

I know you can do it to. Why? Because you bought this book, which means you have invested in yourself, and you want to make a change. So now let's discuss *how* you can make the change.

It is up to you to change your situation, but first, you must say to yourself, "Actually, I'm responsible for my body and my actions. No one is forcing me to overeat, and no one is stopping me from going for a walk." There is no reason not to go for a walk or do some exercise in your home.

Some people blame being too busy on why they're not in shape. It's true that we do lead busy lives, and it can be quite stressful fitting everything in. When I was preparing for my first competition season, I was working full time and commuting for three hours a day. Plus, I was a single parent with two school-age children to look after. I fit everything in, like meal prep and working out, by re-prioritizing things. Some things, like cleaning, just didn't get done. But I never said, "I can't do this, I'm too busy." One of the women being coached by my same coach had an even busier life than I, with three jobs and four children. This made me think, *I'm actually not that busy compared to her*. If you want it badly enough, you will make it work. It's about making *you* the priority and not feeling guilty about it.

You can, for example, get up early to work out or set aside a day to prepare for the coming week. If you're thinking about health and fitness as a priority – and it should be a priority because your family probably relies on you being healthy – it's not selfish. Many women, however, do feel that taking time to eat right and exercise is selfish, but ultimately, it's about health; it's about reducing your risk of cardiovascular disease, stroke, diabetes, and osteoporosis. Looking after your health should be a major priority in your life, along with your family and making a living to pay your bills and keep a roof over your head.

Stress eating generally has to do with masking a feeling. Instead of eating when you're stressed, write down and feel your feelings rather than trying to mask them by eating high fat, sweet, or salty foods. I know that in the short term it gives you that instant fix, but in the long term, it's not helping your health and won't move you forward in any way, shape, or form. It's really important that you identify the feelings and walk through them.

A DOSE OF SELF CONFIDENCE

Building your self-confidence and resilience will also help you reach your goals. If you have an inner voice that tells you, *I am really good at this, I can do this, and I believe in myself,* you're going to be much more likely to be successful than someone who has a negative inner narrative. It's all about having a success and abundance mindset.

Fat loss takes commitment. Can you do this for six to twelve weeks? Can you do it for six months? Can you do it for a year? If you can, you are going to see amazing results. If you can do it for twelve weeks, you're going to see something significant, but the longer that you can commit to this program consistently over time, the greater the rewards will be.

This is something that you don't see in social media; what you see is instant gratification. For example, I post my own before and after pictures, but there's about a five-year difference between them. I'm honest about it, but not everyone is. You may see influencers suggest that you can lose a significant amount of weight in six weeks, but the reality for most people is that it takes a lot longer than that, particularly during and after menopause. If you want to lose weight safely and keep it off for good, slow and steady wins the race.

10 percent of your actions are from the conscious part of your brain, and 90 percent are from the subconscious. When changing your mindset, you need to work on the subconscious part of your brain, and that comes from believing in yourself. It comes from knowing that you're capable, and you're going to be successful.

TIPS FOR CHANGING YOUR SUBCONSCIOUS

Here are some tips on changing your mindset by changing your subconscious.

Start Journaling

Write down your short-term and long-term goals, and the actions that you need to take to achieve those. After you've written them down, repeat them out loud. Treat them like they're positive affirmations.

Think about How You're Going to Approach Fitness

You need to treat this program as seriously as you would your work or business. If you treat it seriously, make the commitment, and give it that energy that you would your job or business, that's when it's going to work for you.

Put Positive Affirmations Around You

Write down the things that drive you or the things you need to do to propel you forward. For example, say, "I am good at working out regularly and sticking to a meal plan," and "I'm also great at sticking to the right calories and macros."

Whatever you're good at, say to yourself; even if you're not good at it yet, you are going to be! Fill in the blank as it applies to you, "I find it easy to..."

If you write that down and say it out loud, it's going to start impacting the subconscious part of your brain. If those negative thoughts start to creep in, try to clear your mind of those and go back to those positive affirmations that you've written down.

Listen to Your Own Voice

I've noticed that the family members or friends of the women I've worked with will put down what they're doing. You need to be quite single minded and not listen to what other people say if you use the approach in this book. Other people will say things like, "You should do keto," "You should do more cardio," or "You should try intermittent fasting." There will always be somebody whose viewpoint will be different than what I have written here, so you've got to block those comments out and trust the process. Most people who are saying this stuff are not qualified to do so and they have not found success with transforming their own body in the long term. Trust the process will work for you and be consistent over time.

Looking after your health in the short and long term and making *you* a priority is really going to help you get through the challenges around you. When my children were younger and I was in my marriage, I put everyone else before me, but in order to get into the right mindset, it was important that I started putting myself first. It might seem a little bit selfish to you and maybe even the people around you, but it's going to benefit everyone in your life if you are the *best* and healthiest version of yourself.

You really need to get out of the mindset that spending time on your body, whether that's training, getting enough sleep, de-stressing, or preparing nutritious food is selfish. It's not selfish; it's being responsible and taking care of your health.

If you've got a partner, and you feel fitter and healthier, that's going to benefit them. It's going to benefit your family because you're going to have more energy, and you're going to live a longer, healthier life. So, you taking care of yourself and putting your needs first is really going to benefit everyone around you.

DON'T FOCUS ON THE END RESULT

So many women come to me and say, "I've been doing this for three weeks, and there's nothing happening. I must be doing something wrong – am I eating right? Am I exercising in the right way?"

If you're consistent with exercise and food, you're going to start to see results, unless you've got some kind of medical problem that prevents it, but you're not going to start seeing results in the first three weeks. Maybe you follow someone on social media, or you know someone who already does this that you trust. Modeling yourself after their behavior can really help. Look at what they're doing right. Typically, they're being consistent over time and not making excuses when it comes to training or nutrition. They're likely also eating the right meals and preparing them in advance.

When you're older, losing fat and building muscle takes time. You shouldn't focus all your time on the end result but instead focus on the process.

Are you being consistent with your food? Are you getting your meal prep done? Are you regularly working out as I described in this book? These are process goals. Make sure you are delivering on those.

Fall in love with the process! If you can enjoy the process and start to celebrate small achievements like a week of eating the right foods and improving in your strength gains, the results will surely follow that. But it is not healthy, and it isn't the right mindset to make progress and be consistent over time if you are constantly jumping on the scale or looking in the mirror saying, "When am I going to see a change?"

MINDSET AND THE POWER OF POSITIVE THINKING

I believe that the power of positive thinking really helps in terms of my own transformation journey, and I've started teaching this to women because many of them have a persistent, negative inner dialogue.

Don't get me wrong – there are some good reasons for feeling this way. You're going through a time in your life where you have become invisible, which usually occurs in your forties and fifties. As you age and notice grey hair and wrinkles, you feel less desirable. You perhaps feel like you're losing both your attractiveness and your identity. You go through a bit of a midlife crisis and can feel quite negative about life. Additionally, as we discussed previously, menopause causes a lot of anxiety and depression; there are legitimate medical reasons due to hormone imbalances that can cause you to think negatively about yourself.

But conversely, this is a time in your life when you can make a positive change and embrace aging and reflect on some of the things that get better when you're older. I don't know about you, but I care less these days about what other people think and do more of what pleases me. I am more open minded about doing something I may have never experienced before. Getting older is a great time to reflect on your life and get rid of what doesn't serve you anymore. You have a lot more knowledge and experience about life, and personally, I feel a lot more comfortable in my own skin. Take time to reflect on the positive aspects of getting older and celebrate the dawning of a new era.

I am a huge believer in the power of positive thinking. I wouldn't have written this book if I wasn't. Thinking positively works well for all aspects of your life, but it works exceptionally well for weight loss, fitness, and health. I don't pretend to have all the knowledge and experience of concepts like the law of attraction and cosmic ordering, but they're really all about the power of positive thinking.

Put your goal in your mind's eye. I thought of myself getting up on stage in a sparkly bikini, but that won't be everyone's goal. It could be getting into your favorite dress or wearing a swimsuit for the first time in a long time. It could be climbing the stairs without getting out of breath. Whatever it is, you need to visualize it and write it down.

You want your vision to be strong and powerful, so close your eyes and imagine your goal. Take a moment, write it down, and make a point to visualize that goal every day. You can do this whenever you like – you may do it first thing in the morning or just before you go to bed at night. Anytime is fine, just make sure to do your visualization when it's quiet, so you can really focus. The location can be anywhere – when you're waiting in your car or when you're taking a walk. Just make it a time that works for you.

If you have an object, it can also help you visualize. If you have a garment you'd like to get into, like a swim-suit, hold on to it while you're picturing it. For exam-ple, I've sent my client a pair of shorts that she's seen me in, and she told me that she would like to get into them herself one day. I've sent those shorts to her in her goal size, so that she can hang them in her closet and visualize herself wearing them.

Once you start visualizing your goals and believing they're possible, you're that much closer to achieving them. I believe, because you've bought this book, you really want to achieve your goal. Now it's about putting everything into practice that you've read here and getting out there and believing in yourself and then achieving it.

SEVEN STEPS TO IMPROVING YOUR MINDSET

When I transformed my body, yes, I had to eat the right food, and yes, I had to exercise, but the key to my success was changing my mindset. Once I did that, everything started to fall into place. Some of these main points will be a recap for you, but know they are so, so important to the end goal of a mindset shift that will take you to the next level.

Find Your Strong Reason Why

I touched upon this earlier and I want to emphasize it again. Explore the reason for wanting to transform your body. Perhaps your transformation is for health reasons, or you just want to look better. I'm in my fifties now and I want longevity. When I get into my sixties, seventies, and eighties, I don't want to be frail; I want to be able to do the things that I enjoy. I want to be really healthy, fit and in fantastic shape now and in the future. Like me, you should want to prevent serious health conditions like heart disease, stroke, and cancer.

If you're healthy now, it will help you prevent some of the serious health problems later in life. You will be able to enjoy your old age with a greater quality of life.

Have you ever heard the term "health is wealth?" You too might want to get into a smaller dress or swimsuit – a lot of women I talk to want to feel good about looking in the mirror. You might have more than one reason for getting fit. Whatever your strong reasons why, write them down – writing them down makes them more likely to happen. There is scientific evidence that shows this is the case.

Make Yourself a Priority and Love Yourself

So many women who I come across do not prioritize their own health above everyone else's. Does that sound familiar? If it does, then you've got to start making yourself a priority because all your loved ones are going to benefit. Remember, as women, we are poor at making ourselves a priority, but you shouldn't feel that you're being selfish or shy away from taking care of your appearance and wanting to look good. Improving your health will also improve your mental health at a time when you may be suffering more from anxiety and depression.

My goodness, when I transformed my body, boy did I feel so good about myself! With my new-found confidence I entered and won bikini competitions, found a new life partner, and started to help others get in shape. But I did this by making myself a priority.

This is a form of self-love. Reflect on this. Do you love yourself? Answer this question honestly. If you don't love yourself, it's highly likely that no one else will. Part of self-love is believing you are deserving of good things happening to you and that you deserve to take time out for yourself to be the *best* version of yourself.

Form Good Daily Habits and Kick the Bad Ones

You can change your habits by getting into a really good routine. This does require motivation, planning, and discipline at first, but then you just do it without thinking. Take hand washing for example. Prior to COVID I remember going in public bathrooms and witnessing people not washing their hands. But now *everyone* washes their hands driven by the fact that it will help prevent the spread of COVID and other viruses. In fact, we are meticulous about washing our hands not only after the bathroom but also after going out anywhere. That has now become a habit that you don't even have to think about; you just do it.

For example, you can remove items from your home that encourage your bad habits, like high fat, high salt, and high sugar foods. You can put workout equipment and walking shoes in a visible place. One of the things I need to do every day is get on the foam roller, so it's staring me in the face in my bedroom where I'm much more likely to use it. I never put it away. Keep some chopped salad in the fridge for you to snack on if you get the munchies (that's not hunger, by the way). Get your meals prepped in advance so that if you are hungry, your next meal is within easy reach. Make the good habits easy and make the bad habits more difficult.

Take Responsibility

To reiterate what I said earlier, it's easy to blame others for the situation you are in. I have heard phrases like "the pandemic made me this way," or "I can't lose weight because I'm in menopause." I know those things can make you gain weight and can make it difficult to lose weight, but if you've consumed more food or been less active than you should have, you need to take responsibility for your actions.

People who are in great shape have the right mindset – they acknowledge if they have been eating badly or not exercising enough and don't blame outside forces. If you are not in the shape you would like to be, it's down to you, isn't it? No one is force feeding you or physically stopping you from exercising.

Work on Self-Belief

Years ago, I didn't have much confidence, but when I started to believe in myself, things started to change for me. Now I can't give you self-belief, but you can write down the things that you are good at and start to change your inner narrative. Start to talk yourself up, saying things like, *I can do this, I can achieve it*. If you start to believe in yourself a bit, more great things will happen, I promise.

Make a Commitment and Write It Down

Keep a journal of what you're doing. For example, when you say it yourself, *I am going to work out three times a week,* put it down on paper or make a digital note. As I said earlier, writing things down makes them more likely to happen. If your goal is weight or fat loss, write down how you're going to achieve that – what are you going to do? For instance, are you going to purchase a meal plan or are you going to track your calories and macros through an app? You need to set out an action plan of *exactly* what you are going to do to achieve your goals. You can't just say, "I want to lose weight." It won't work. If you make that commitment and write it down in detail with goal dates attached, you're much more likely to do it.

Remember the Power of Positive Thinking

The power of positive thinking does link a little bit to what I said about self-belief. You need to visualize something to believe it, then achieve it. The mind is such a powerful thing. If you believe things are going in your favor, it's more likely to happen. If you've read this far, you really want this, don't you? Start thinking positively. Think about what you can do, what you've achieved so far, and think about what you're going to achieve and start to play it out in your mind. What are you going to look like? What dress size will you be? How healthy will you be? Close your eyes and spend time each day to start to visualize what that's going to look like. Use the power of your mind, and things will start to happen for you.

THE POWER OF SUPPORT IN YOUR TRANSFORMATION JOURNEY

Many people find that changing their mindset is a challenging endeavor, especially when attempted alone. The journey to transform your body and mind requires consistent effort, resilience, and a strong support system. This is why many who participate in my challenges or watch my YouTube videos eventually choose to work with me as private coaching clients. Having a coach provides the guidance, accountability, and encouragement necessary to navigate the ups and downs of this transformative journey. It's not a sign of weakness to seek support; in fact, recognizing the need for guidance and taking action to get it is a testament to your strength and commitment.

Through private coaching, I've witnessed countless women achieve their goals by leveraging the power of a personalized approach and a supportive community. They find solace in knowing they are not alone and that someone is there to guide them through every step of the process. This support system helps reinforce the mindset shifts needed to sustain long-term success, turning potential setbacks into opportunities for growth. If you're struggling to make these changes on your own, consider seeking the support you deserve – it might just be the key to unlocking your fullest potential.

As we come to the final chapter of this book, remember that the journey to better health, fitness, and a positive mindset is ongoing. It's not about achieving perfection but about making consistent, meaningful progress. You've learned about the importance of strength training, nutrition, rest, and mindset. Now, it's time to put these pieces together and create the life you've always envisioned.

Change is never easy, but with determination, the

right strategies, and a supportive network, you can overcome any obstacle. Embrace the process, celebrate your victories, and learn from your challenges. Your transformation is within reach, and by applying the knowledge and tools provided in this book, you are well on your way to becoming the best version of yourself. Believe in your strength, trust the journey, and take that first step towards a healthier, happier you.

11

YOUR SECOND ACT – EMBRACING A STRONGER YOU

R emember Linda from Chapter 1? Our beautiful, fifty-two-year-old mom who stood frustrated in front of her closet, feeling disconnected from herself? That Linda – the one who was so skilled at shoving her monster just a little deeper into the closet each day – is a distant memory now. After going through the steps I have laid out in this book, Linda shed seventeen pounds and an impressive six inches off her waist in just eight weeks by taking part in my 8-week Transformation Challenge.

Linda's transformation didn't end with my 8-week transformation challenge. She's continually setting new goals, both physical and mental. You'll often find her with a self-help book in hand, seeking ways to grow and improve. Her confidence has soared, and her mental resilience has become as impressive as her physical strength.

The impact on her family has been profound, as her newfound energy and confidence rippled through her family life. Linda's daughter, Zoe, now joins her for workouts, learning valuable lessons about health and self-care. Her husband, Kevin, has been an unwavering source of support, cheering her on every step of the way.

Perhaps most inspiring is Linda's shift in perspective. She's no longer just working out to fit into old clothes; she's "training for her ninety-year-old self," focusing on long-term health and vitality. This commitment to continual self-improvement has created a ripple effect, inspiring friends and family to embark on their own wellness journeys.

Linda's story isn't unique – it represents the potential for change that exists in you. She shows that with the right mindset, support, and tools, transformation is not only possible but also sustainable.

WILL YOU ACCEPT THE CHALLENGE?

When it comes to menopause and weight loss for women over forty, you should never just consider being in a calorie deficit. You must manage the five main areas that we've covered in this book – how much protein you take in (balancing it with carbohydrates and fats), eating for your hormones, building muscle through strength training, and focusing on getting good quality sleep and continually working on your mindset.

It is equally important to reduce your stress levels because it's hard to lose weight if you're stressed. Stress, as we've covered in earlier chapters, wreaks havoc on your hormones.

When working through the plans I've covered here, you'll need to remember this lifestyle doesn't come easy, which is why you need to have the right mindset. Beginning this program takes dedication; it takes hard work as well as rest, so make sure that you give yourself one to two days a week when you're not doing strenuous exercise. I would encourage you to continue using this book as a guide for your physical and mental transformation.

Surely remember the old saying, "Insanity is doing the same thing over and over and expecting different results." I was two years into my journey when I had my epiphany. I had worked in several programs with different trainers (who mostly focused on the wrong training and only focused on a calorie deficit), spent considerable amounts of time and money, and still had not seen any real results.

When I decided to go back to lifting heavy, which had worked for me before, I started to look more closely at my nutrition and focused on old school bodybuilder methods, like consuming high amounts of protein because I knew I wanted to build muscle. When I started to research further, I realized that muscle burns fat. So, I developed a nutrition plan around that idea.

I'll admit, I didn't get it absolutely perfect straight-away. There was a lot of trial and error; I looked for quick fixes, and I wasn't always eating correctly before training. But I soon learned, especially after deciding to compete in bodybuilding competitions, how to get my nutrition dialed in. I discovered that what I ate was going to make a big difference in how I could transform my body.

If you can follow the path that I've outlined here, I have no doubt that it will work for you, but it's going to require a considerable commitment over time. It may take months or even a year for you to see real results. You'll need to have the discipline to work out and regularly stick to a meal plan.

There are no quick fixes. This program requires patience because women over forty take longer to lose body fat than any other demographic. I talk to women in the bodybuilding community, and they are well aware how much harder it is for us to lose body fat than it is for younger women. It's simply going to take us longer to lose weight and put on muscle. But that muscle is the thing that's going to help us burn fat.

If you have that commitment, discipline, and patience, you'll see results from everything I've shared with you in this book. If you want to find out more, visit my website and download my free plan at melissaneill.com/plan, social media pages and my app, but if you begin with just the information I've laid out here, you'll go in the right direction.

I wish you the best of luck on your fitness journey and remember – this isn't a quick fix. It's a lifestyle.

ACKNOWLEDGMENTS

For many years, the community of women that follow me on YouTube and other social media platforms have said to me, "You ought to write a book." That's what first sowed the seed in my mind. I'd like to thank my community of Strong Women who made me believe in myself enough that if I wrote a book, they would actually read it!

A special thanks goes to Michelle Nati, who helped me put together the first draft of this book. Michelle is a client of mine and was invaluable in the early stages when putting together this book.

A *huge* thanks goes out to my partner, Kennedy Charles, a tower of strength and support, who when I come up with these crazy ideas is 100 percent behind me. Without him, I could never have built this growing empire and helped thousands of women to achieve their dream body.

My family, Luke, Laura, Frits, Joan, Flynn, and Yas have shown me tremendous support and continue to be a source of inspiration for my storytelling and drive to be the best person I can possibly be.

I want to thank my team at Body By Bikini, who have been a consistent source of support, ideas, and inspiration.

And thank you to Angela Lauria at The Author Incubator, who helped turn my dream of becoming an author into a reality.

ABOUT THE AUTHOR

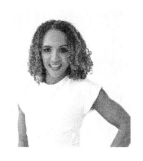 Melissa Neill is a YouTuber and fitness coach helping women over forty transform their bodies. She is the founder and CEO of Body By Bikini fitness and weight loss programs specifically designed for women over forty. She has helped over 10,000 women through her Body By Bikini app and personal coaching work to break through menopause and achieve their dream body and health.

Melissa is also a mother of three children. Born in 1967, after spending her early years in Ghana, Melissa moved to the UK at age six. She was educated at Fairfield Grammar School but left school at sixteen without completing her formal education. She later returned to education and achieved a first-class honors degree at the University of the West of England in 1991. Melissa has twenty-five plus years working in the public relations industry, including the healthcare sector.

Having found a lack of information on weight loss for women over forty and going through menopause, in 2019, Melissa decided to set up her own YouTube channel. In June 2020, Melissa led her first online fitness and weight loss program for women over forty and is the first in her industry to do this solely for this age group in her own app, Body By Bikini. At the time of writing Body By Bikini has received 40,000 plus app downloads and over 10,000 women enrolled into one of the programs.

Since she began her own business, Melissa has helped thousands of women with her unique method of weight loss, involving weightlifting and high protein eating. She also holds regular live Masterclasses that educate women around the time of menopause on fitness, health, and weight loss. Melissa has also been featured on Good Morning America, taken part in podcasts, and featured in magazine articles. You can find out more at melissaneill.com.

At the time of writing, she has over 300,000-plus subscribers and 37 million-plus views on YouTube, plus 60k followers on Instagram and 170k followers on TikTok. Melissa's no nonsense and relatable approach has helped inform thousands of menopausal women about how to get in shape when they reach this difficult stage in their lives.

Melissa also enjoys competing in bodybuilding shows, having competed in five, taking home twelve trophies including three first places and two pro cards (for Elite status athletes). Melissa lives with her partner and two of her children in the South West of England.

GIFT FOR READER

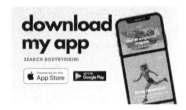

Dear Strong Woman,

Thank you for purchasing this book. It takes real courage to take back control of your health – especially as a woman during menopause.

I'm here to show you that your dream body is not only possible – but it's well within reach.

I am living proof at fifty-seven years old, and so are the 10,000+ women I've helped who are in their forties, fifties, sixties – and beyond.

To show you just how grateful I am for your commitment, I want to **give you my signature 7-Day Plan for free.**

Start losing inches in weeks and finally get the body you want!

Here's what's included in my 7-Day Plan:

- Mindset Training
- Strength Training Guide
- Lower Body Weight Workout
- Upper Body Weight Workout
- Full Body Gym Workout
- 16-Minute HIIT Workout
- Meal Schedule and Ideas for Meat Eaters
- Plant-Based Meal Schedule and Ideas for Vegans.

I've put this plan together as the perfect way to kickstart your journey and get your momentum going with everything you have learned in this book.

All you have to do is go to melissaneill.com/plan and start your no-commitment, 7-day free trial.

You won't be charged once the 7 days are complete – you don't even give your payment details. This is just to give you access to the plan. It's yours FREE forever!

I know this is going to be the best way to begin your new chapter. And trust me, we are just getting started.

Here's to you looking and feeling your best – no matter what your age!

Lots of Love,

Melissa X